W9-CHS-286

NO MORE DIETING!

PERMANENT WEIGHT LOSS WITHOUT DIETING AND FREEDOM FROM COMPULSIVE EATING

SHAUNA COLLINS, MD

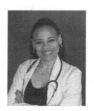

NO MORE DIETING!

Updated May 2019

Copyright © 2016 All Rights Reserved

All rights reserved. No part of this publication may be reproduced, distributed, or transmitted in any form or by any means, including photocopying, recording, or other electronic or mechanical methods, without the prior written permission of the publisher, except in the case of brief quotations embodied in reviews and certain other non-commercial uses permitted by copyright law.

ISBN-13:978-1541268098
ISBN-10:1541268091

FREE AUDIO DOWNLOAD!

READ THIS FIRST

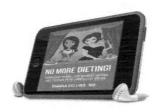

Thank you for purchasing *No More Dieting!*
To show my appreciation,
I would like to give you the gift of a FREE audio download of
The Essentials of No More Dieting!

Which includes:
7 Mindset Principles (*MIND*) and
4 Action Steps (*MOTION*)

TO DOWNLOAD GO TO:
www.NoMoreDieting.com/freegift

DEDICATION

∾

*To my patients and all who struggle
with overeating and suffer from obesity*

I wrote this book for you.

You will find freedom within these pages.

THANK YOU

~

To God for *everything*.

To my Honey, Demetric: Undoubtedly, you are God's gift to me. You are the rock that keeps me grounded in the cyclone that sometimes (well, usually) is our life. Thank you for your never-ending patience as I brainstorm (and execute) endlessly. Thank you for allowing me to be me. I am so grateful for you! I love you forever.

Joshua and Daniel: Thank you just for being my babies! Your very existence fuels my soul with continuous joy and motivates me to be the best I can. Thank you for your patience throughout the many days I had to give my attention to this project instead of you. I hope you know that you're central to the reason I work as hard as I do. I love you deeply.

Mom: I love you. You taught me what *love in action* looks like without ever saying a word. I wouldn't be the mother I am and strive to be if I didn't have you as my example. There aren't enough "thank yous."

Stephen: Thank you for your wise counsel, your love, and your endless support. Thank you for all the years of making me laugh until I cry. You're the best brother God could've given me! I love you Broham!

Jaimie: JB, thank you for decades of spiritual counseling, tireless prayers, and for your love and support. I don't think I'd be the person I am today had you not been my sister. I love you Liver! Here's leg to ya!

Sonya (the Biz Wiz): Sonya, There's so much I enjoy about you and that I've learned from you over the years. I'm so grateful to have you as a sister! I love you.

SuszeeQ: My dear cousin, you are a priceless gift from God in my life and have always been. I'm so grateful for all the years God has allowed us to journey through together! I thank you and Leon for all that you do and for your immeasurable generosity. I love you QD and Neon!

Fe: Thank you for decades of sisterhood. No price can be placed on such a friendship. I love you Febe! My life is enriched because you are in it.

Jovanna and Shondia: Thank you for allowing me to share in your life. I am blessed to be able to call each of you *daughter*. I love you both.

To All the Babes: Bryson, Jordi, Summer, Savannah (babygirl), Aasha, Matai, Vanessa, Savannah (ladygirl). Life provides us the extraordinary opportunity to do just about anything we want with it. Be wise and make good use of it! I'm expecting to hear great things. I love you. You're always in my prayers.

Sijara, Susie2, and the homeschool moms: You all have touched my life in a multitude of ways. I cherish our friendship and fellowship!

Lise Cartwright: Thank you for helping me pull it all together! Your expertise, organization, and just the right amount of *cracking that whip* was exactly what I needed to birth my vision and bring it to life. Thank you!

Chandler Bolt and Self-Publishing School: Although I had the resolve to publish for years, SPS gave me the *'how to'* that I was missing. Thank you Chandler and all those at SPS!

TABLE OF CONTENTS

MEDICATION

MY STORY AND THE BIRTH OF NO MORE DIETING!

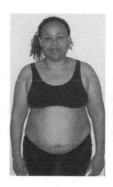 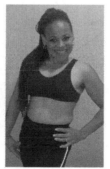

Left: Dr. Collins After 30 Years of Dieting
Right: Dr. Collins After 6 Months of No More Dieting!

"Wow! You look great!"

Kay looked me up and down with her eyes popping out of her head. I hadn't seen her in a while, and she was used to seeing me much bigger.

"What diet are you doing? You have to tell me!"

"No diet," I said. I think her eyes got even bigger. "I don't diet anymore. I refuse to diet anymore."

Kay looked bewildered. "I don't get it. So how did you lose the weight?"

Kay knew all about my lifetime struggle with food and weight, as I knew about hers. She was aware that as an obese child, I was taken to my first fat clinic at age 7, prescribed a handful of pills to take multiple times a day, and got a shot in the rump twice a week to boot.

Naturally, I protested and my mom eventually took me out of the program. I remained that fat kid for several years until I became anorexic at thirteen. I would allow myself only water for two days then eat on the third day, then repeat. This resulted in a fifty-pound weight loss over one school semester.

But one day I ate and couldn't stop eating. Determined not to gain all my weight back, I began vomiting up the food. This marked a nine-year stretch of bulimia, which I practiced multiple times a day.

Finally, at twenty-two, I'd had enough. With the help of family,

I was admitted into an inpatient recovery unit where I stopped the binge-purge cycle – at least for the thirty days I was there. I relapsed upon discharge, but I remained in counseling and attended regular recovery meetings. It was touch and go for a while as I struggled to live 'normal' in the outside world. Eventually, I remained abstinent from bulimia but continued binge-eating. I promptly ballooned back to a state of obesity, and there I remained for the next twenty years.

Kay and I knew each other through mutual friends. All of us gals would get together at one of our homes every so often. Kay and I would inevitably migrate to each other and bond over exchanging our 'fat chick' woes. We'd discuss our love for food, our most recent bingecapades, and empathize with each other as fellow food addicts. We'd wrap up our discussion by deciding to do the latest diet together, starting tomorrow (always tomorrow), so we could finally become the divas that we knew we were meant to be.

Then we'd celebrate our upcoming gorgeousness with the yummy eats we all brought to girls night. Sort of a last supper type of feast. When we'd see each other a few months later, we'd both be just as big, same as always, and we'd launch into our fat chick sagas again, same as always. It was like a bad recurring dream that carried on for years.

So you can imagine Kay's surprise when she saw me this time around. I was no longer wearing double-digit sizes, my face was chiseled, and my belly was flat (well, flatter anyway). I looked fabulous and felt amazing! I had arrived at the destination we both had dreamed of our whole lives. Yet I was telling her that dieting had nothing to do with it! She was utterly baffled.

I said to her, "Sit down, girl. I can't wait to break it down to you!"

Kay dropped like an anchor onto the couch and I landed right beside her. We tuned out the other girls. She was all ears and I was eager to share...

It all started during my last year in medical school. I had given birth to my second son several months earlier. I was already obese when I got pregnant, and now I was stuck with an additional forty pounds that I hadn't lost after giving birth. I was beyond huge! I felt like a big, fat pastry. A soft, doughy, amorphous blob bumbling about, all short of breath in my plus-size clothes. Gross. Just gross. I was so embarrassed.

I had never been content being obese, but I had been the same weight (give or take a few pounds) for about twenty years. So I had adapted and became somewhat comfortable with my size. I was big, but I maximized my cuteness in the skin I was in, and life went on. But now I was outside of my comfort zone. Waaaay outside of my comfort zone. I couldn't even pull off fat-cute anymore. Now I was just fat! I couldn't take it. I had gone too far.

I was doing a medical rotation in Northridge, California when I found myself standing frozen in the midst of the cafeteria at lunchtime. I looked around at all the options and wondered for the millionth time 'Ok. What do I eat? Hot food? No, looks too greasy. Deli? Maybe. The salad bar perhaps? No, not feeling it. But I do need to find something low-cal.

Actually, low-cal and low-carb. It should be high protein too. Yeah, low-cal, low-carb, high protein. That's how I really should eat if I'm going to be a good girl today. How about a snack? Hmmmm...maybe one of those 100-calorie snack packs? No. I hate those. I can eat 10 of those. One is just a tease.

How about fruit instead? Yeah, fruit. Oh, but then I'm not low-carb anymore. Well, that depends on the fruit and how much of it I eat...aww forget it! Too much to think about! I'll just grab something to drink.

Hmmmm...what to drink, what to drink? Diet soda? No, I really should cut back and drink more water. But I don't want water. Maybe flavored water? Or how about a diet Snapple? That's kind of a compromise...or is it?...' and on and on and on it went.

I suddenly became aware that I felt tired. So tired. Exhausted really. So I just sat down. I thought about the infinite food choices and I thought about my weight. I was determined to take the extra weight off, but how? I just couldn't figure out what to do!

Over the years, I tried to follow the dieting trends and the official recommendations. But no matter what I did, I failed at losing weight time and time again. Why did it all have to be so complicated?

In my usual mode of desperation, I considered dieting yet again, because it was all I knew. Then out of nowhere, something inside of me screamed, *"No more dieting! Don't fool your-*

self! You know dieting doesn't work! Don't waste another second on it!"

This was something I had never experienced before. It was like I was being shaken to my senses from the inside out!

In an instant I resolved to never resort to dieting again. Just like that the door slammed shut to the option of dieting. It was locked once and for all and I knew at that moment I would never go back. This was exciting! But I was apprehensive as well.

So what now? If dieting isn't the answer, how am I going to get the weight off? I began considering a few simple concepts.

What if I...

freely allow myself to eat whenever I'm genuinely hungry? No more enduring hours of starvation like I did when I was dieting.

And what if I...

allowed myself to eat whatever I wanted? As long as I made it a point to **stop** eating at the earliest sign that my body (not my taste buds, or my emotions) was satisfied.

But I really should try to...

eat only if and when I am genuinely hungry - instead of eating just for the sake of eating as I've always done before. This would mean no stress eating or self-medicating with food. No boredom eating or unconscious TV snacking without any thought as to whether or not I am even hungry.

Hmm...*disciplined liberty*. I like it. I like it a lot. Sort of the 'ol eat to live, don't live to eat approach. Feels natural. Normal. But could I do it? Could I practice such discipline?

I had always considered myself *uncontrollable* when it came to eating. Especially with eating foods that I love. Dare I now consider living so freely? Living with no lists of foods that I can and cannot eat? Could I be trusted with such freedom?

It seemed pretty audacious! But I loved the idea of eating from a place of authenticity for a change. Eating with consideration as to what my body may actually want or need, rather than just trying to manipulate it with diets for the sake of weight loss.

Yes! I can do this! It's totally reasonable, it makes perfect sense!

From this day forward...

- I'll eat whenever I'm truly hungry. No starving allowed!
- When I'm truly hungry and I'm ready to eat, I will eat whatever I want! There will be no restrictions in my food choices. No deprivation. But I will strive to make healthy choices as often as I can.
- I'll do my best to stop eating once my body is satisfied and I no longer feel hungry. I won't eat to satisfy my emotions. I'll try to stop at the point when I feel pressure in my belly, not when I have to unbutton my pants.
- I won't eat during the hours that I'm not genuinely

hungry. If I have no sign of hunger, such as a gnawing, empty feeling in my gut or a growling stomach, I will hold off on eating until I do.

And with this, the basic framework of *No More Dieting* was born.

Sitting in the hospital cafeteria, I asked myself, so what do I *really* want to eat for lunch? Numerous possibilities ran through my mind. Of all the options I considered, it was an egg salad sandwich that I desired that day. Quite anticlimactic, I know, but authentic nonetheless. I knew it was a sincere desire because it made my mouth water when I thought of eating it. So egg salad sandwich for lunch it would be!

Next, instead of grabbing a pre-made sandwich and enhancing it with gobs of mayonnaise (yes, I'm one of those), I considered what I could do to enjoy the taste I wanted, but in the healthiest way possible. I decided to construct my own egg salad sandwich. I grabbed six boiled eggs, kept all the whites but just one yolk.

Instead of using three or four packets of mayo, I used only one and added a little mustard, salt, and pepper. I ate the egg salad on one slice of wheat bread, along with an apple, and a bottle of water.

I was shocked when I noticed a sense of fullness in my gut after this small meal (well, small to me anyway), and I was totally amazed that I was completely satisfied! Egg salad? Really? Who would've known!

I left the cafeteria with a bounce in my step. Although I had just eaten, I felt lighter walking out than I had coming in. For the first time in, well, ever, I felt like I was in control. In control of my food, in control of myself, and in control of my life. A pretty big boost in confidence for just one lunchtime victory, but I knew I was on to something. This was the beginning of greater things to come!

I promised myself I would not eat again until my stomach actually growled, indicating for sure that I was truly hungry. When it growled, I ate again, but not before.

Each time I ate, I asked myself beforehand what was it that I truly wanted to eat. My choices ran the gamut from salad to cake, from fruit to chocolate, from beef to fish, and everything in between. I ate it all and loved every bite! And to my delight, the weight began coming off!

What was equally fulfilling, if not more, was the increase in self-esteem and morale I developed as I learned to trust myself with my desires, while simultaneously respecting the boundaries of my body. The more I trusted myself to eat authentically, the stronger I became and the more I actually enjoyed practicing discipline.

In hindsight, this makes sense. People tend to want to live up to the trust that's granted them, but they may also live up to the distrust that's ascribed to them, albeit unintentionally. I hadn't realized that the lack of faith I had in myself to manage my behavior and the needs of my body was like a perpetual, self-fulfilling prophesy!

Enthusiastically, I shared all of this with Kay. I wrapped up my narrative by explaining to her that the well-thought-out egg salad sandwich marked the beginning of effortless weight loss for me and true freedom from compulsive eating.

But Kay had only one question. "How long have you been doing this and how much weight have you lost?"

I was a little taken aback. I had raved all about literally having my cake and eating it too and the joy of eating authentically. I spoke of so many amazing benefits, not just physical, but psychological as well.

Frankly, I was surprised (and a little perturbed) that my weight loss was all she was interested in after everything I had shared. Nevertheless, I stammered, "Uh, it's been about five months and I've lost thirty pounds."

She didn't look impressed. Maybe I didn't explain it right. "That's six dress sizes on me!" I added to emphasize my achievement.

She scoffed, almost snorted. "That's only six pounds a month! I can lose that in a week!"

That was it. Case dismissed.

I was stunned. I looked at her in awe and disbelief. It was as though she hadn't heard anything else I had said. The only thing that mattered was how much weight I had lost and in how much time. She couldn't appreciate the breadth of the healing and restoration I was trying to relay.

I realized that Kay was still in the mindset of looking for the ever-elusive *quick fix*. She was waiting for the next *abracadabra diet* that promises "30 pounds lost in 30 days…or your money back!" I understood this mindset all too well because this had been me just 5 months earlier.

I immediately felt grateful to be on the other side of this futile thinking. But I was disappointed that I was unable to successfully convey the freedom and peace that occurs when we give up trying to live within the constraints of dieting and instead eat and live from a place of authenticity. Kay was having no part of it. She was still chasing the dream, looking for that miracle weight loss solution.

Although I sensed defeat, I gave it one last shot. "It doesn't have to take five months. That's just how long it took me. But even if it does, how many times has five months passed by without having lost the weight? And at least this way, the weight is lost easily! It's lost without dieting, so it's painless! There's no torture!"

Crickets.

Girl, bye.

~

Over the next year or two, I saw Kay a few more times. She continued to complain about all the weight she needed to lose. I offered to walk her through the process of real change, but she wasn't interested. Instead, she would say things like, "I'm glad it worked for you. But I can't allow myself to eat my binge foods! I can't control myself! I'd gain 100 more pounds!"

"No Kay," I'd say. "You binge on those foods *because you don't allow yourself to have them.* If they weren't off-limits, they would lose their appeal and wouldn't seem like such a big deal. After having them freely a few times, you wouldn't want them as often." I told her that by fixing the problem on the inside (namely her perspective) the outside would naturally follow. But I was never able to convince her. She eventually moved away, and we lost touch.

I realized then that the counseling I offer will not be received by everyone. It's not tangible like a case of diet food that can readily be hauled away from a clinic. And it requires more participation than just passively being told how many calories to consume or what type of food to eat in order to lose weight. These actions seem easier to embrace because the dieter gets to place (or *misplace*) the responsibility of change onto something outside of themselves. Denial shades the truth; buying false hope and comfort for a while.

No More Dieting **calls for active introspection and elimination of unprofitable beliefs followed by action.**

Everyone is not up to the task of taking charge of their life in this way. But for those of you who sense that permanent change comes from the inside-out, I invite you to jump off the hamster wheel of dieting and join me on the path of true transformation.

Are you ready?

Of course you are.

Now let's go...

MIND

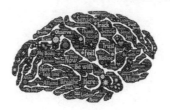

THE 7 NO MORE DIETING
MINDSET PRINCIPLES FOR PERMANENT WEIGHT LOSS

MIND

INTRODUCTION

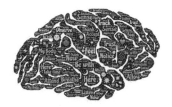

There are 7 *No More Dieting* Mindset Principles

Since all change first begins in the mind, this is the place where our journey begins.

Here in **MIND** we will discuss changing our perspective to develop a healthy mindset that will take us from perpetual bondage and defeat in our eating to a place of peace and liberation.

Make sure you're in a place where distractions are minimal and you can peacefully delve into this teaching. If you are not at this moment, that's fine. Review the principles again once you are. They are not to be rushed and they can't be missed. Absorbing these principles leads to the shift in perspective we need to never struggle with food and weight again.

~

The 7 *No More Dieting* Mindset Principles are listed below. Let's discuss each one in detail.

What Should I Eat?

- Principle #1 Eat What You Authentically Want
- Principle #2 Always Strive to Make Healthy Choices

When Should I Eat?

- Principle #3 Eat Whenever You Are Truly Hungry
- Principle #4 Stop Eating As Soon As Your Body Is Satisfied (not your taste buds, or your emotional state)
- Principle #5 Don't Eat Again until You're Truly Hungry

My Mindset

- Principle #6 Don't Expect Perfection. Just Do Your Best Each Day!
- Principle #7 Start Today. *Always* Today

WHAT SHOULD I EAT?

MIND

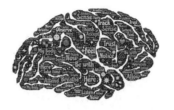

EAT WHAT YOU AUTHENTICALLY WANT!

NMD MINDSET PRINCIPLE #1

There are no food restrictions or *off-limit* foods.

Food restriction of some sort is the foundation of most diets. By imposing dietary restrictions, we mistakenly think (or hope) that these rules and regulations will somehow keep us from overeating. But the result is quite the opposite!

Like strapping into a straitjacket, dietary restrictions produce the urge within us to escape their constraints and be set free again.

The moment we begin to diet, inner pressure begins building like water behind a dam and we begin to long for the foods we have made off-limits. Longing gradually turns into obsession, and inner tension continues to rise.

Eventually, the dam gives way and the pressure is relieved, often by binging on the forbidden foods. There is angst and urgency to the binge, like one who is gasping for air after holding their breath for too long. With every bite, tension is relieved and a calm takes over, like the early effect of anesthesia.

But with relief comes pain. Because like a trapped wolf, we chewed off our own foot in order to escape the shackles. Now we have a new problem, or rather an old one. We're back at square one. We gained back all the weight we had lost and then some.

What then do we do? Knowing deep down it can't possibly work, we plan the next failing diet, because restriction is all we know. Round, and round, and round we go...

So what's the solution?

We No Longer Diet and We Don't Restrict

We no longer impose rules and regulations on what we eat, because as you and I have experienced, making food off-limits only creates an obsession for those very foods. This obsession ultimately leads to binging. Mental torment is present throughout the dieting and in the aftermath of the binge as well. This is no way for us to live!

But be encouraged! There is a way to end this mental and physical cycle of destruction. We stop it by abandoning the *don't look, don't touch, don't eat* approach to weight loss. No food is ever off-limits again.

There are no food restrictions (unless prescribed by your doctor due to medical necessity). All food is equally permissible, thus no food is particularly special. Consequently, no food has the psychological lure it did in times past when we labeled it "forbidden" out of fear of abusing it and gaining weight. All food eventually loses its seductive effect.

But Dr. Collins, I'm afraid if I allow myself to eat all my favorite foods, I'll be pigging out on them every day!

This is usually the response I get from patients when I tell them not to restrict what they eat. They panic and exclaim that they *must* eliminate their "binge foods," because every time they eat them, they're not able to stop!

"Well, you're not eating them *now*." Silent pause. I let them mull that over a bit. "So you certainly *must* be able to stop." Blank stare. I have their attention.

I go on to explain that these foods have *become* their binge foods because they decided to restrict them at some point during their dieting days. We want all the more what we can't have. Therefore, the greater the resolve to restrict, *the greater the desire* for that which is restricted.

So despite the many unrestricted foods they allowed on their diet, the focus (and soon obsession) becomes the foods they limited. When they finally eat these coveted foods, they eat them as if there were no tomorrow. They conclude they have no control when eating these foods so they should be avoided at all cost. They believe the only way to lose weight is to make them *completely* off-limits.

But this only fuels the fire of desire and intensifies the obsession, leading to repeated attempts at abstinence and inevitable failures. The process is like a snowball rolling downhill, gaining size, force, and momentum, posing a greater threat with every cyclic rotation.

Seemingly counterintuitive, the truth is that freedom from food obsession and binging comes from *relinquishing* dietary restrictions, not attempting to live within them. Therefore, all foods are permitted.

But if I take the reins completely off, won't I lose control, go buck wild, and roll around naked in pools of chocolate?

You may for a minute. To be honest, I know I did. I ate dessert most days in the beginning of my new-found freedom. But this is a temporary response.

Imagine letting a kid loose in a candy store with no restrictions. The immediate result is predictable. All the years of mom's loving restraint and wise nutritional counsel goes out the door, and the kid goes hog wild. He can't get the treats in his mouth fast enough.

But hold on just a minute. Let's take a look down the road a bit.

How's the kid's behavior on the second day if he's still in the store? If he eats any candy at all, it's very little. He's lost significant interest because physically, his body is signaling "No more sugar please!"

This signaling may manifest as the *absence* of a sense of desire, no mouth-watering, or no stomach growling when he thinks of eating the sweets. Or there may even be an all-out *negative response* such as a sense of *repulsion or nausea* with the thought of eating more candy.

Psychologically, he's losing interest because there's no longer the *forbidden fruit* factor of wanting what he can't have. He can now have as much sugar as he wants, whenever he wants. So, the instinct to grab and eat them as fast as he can before he's restrained again is completely gone. Having free access, they have lost their magic.

Now, what if the kid *lives* in the store, as you and I now live in complete dietary freedom with no restrictions? Living there, he will naturally settle into a dietary balance. He'll still enjoy some goodies now and then, but the *yearning* he had for the sweets back when he was restricted is entirely gone.

Another example:

Picture a kid on Christmas day receiving the toy he asked and hoped for incessantly for weeks and months prior. Now picture that same kid with the same toy a month later. Now 3 months later. How special is that toy 6 months down the line?

Is he even still playing with the toy *at all?*

Eat What You Authentically Desire

When you are truly hungry and thinking about what you should eat, be authentic! Ask yourself, what do I truly want? Ignore the *diet voice* within that suggests only 'diet-foods.' Likewise, ignore the voice of the *binge eater* that will urge you to eat what you previously called your 'binge foods.'

These suggestions come from opposite sides of the same coin. The coin is **fear**. The diet-related suggestion comes from fear of losing control and gaining weight or never losing the weight. The binge-related suggestion comes from fear of scarcity, restriction, and deprivation.

Rather than immediately going with the strongest urge, calmly try to discern what your pure, unadulterated desire is. What food makes your mouth water when you think of eating it at that moment?

Conversely, what food produces no response or a negative response? Follow your body's natural cues and eat the food that will satisfy your true self for that particular meal. It's perfectly fine if it turns out that the food you truly desire to eat happens to be what you previously called a 'diet' or a 'binge' food. If this is what you truly desire to eat, by all means, eat it!

There will be times when you aren't aware of having a desire to eat one particular food over others. Or, sometimes food options are limited and the opportunity to choose may not exist. No problem! The point here isn't about *what* we eat. It's to learn to eat from a place of *authenticity* rather than a sense of bondage and fear.

As for me, my daily dessert fest inevitably ceased. Now I mainly just eat desserts when they are present at an event I'm attending or I may purchase them myself once or twice a month. I still adore sweets, but they've lost their irresistible allure. The obsession for them is gone because I know I can have them whenever I want.

And so it will be with you as you lift food restrictions and learn to eat according to your body's natural cues and your authentic desire.

～

Summary of NMD Principle #1
Eat What You Authentically Want!

We abandon dieting once and for all. We have no food restrictions (unless medically indicated). No foods are off-limits. We strive daily to eat naturally, according to our authentic desires.

ALWAYS STRIVE TO MAKE HEALTHY CHOICES!

NMD MINDSET PRINCIPLE #2

*E*liminating all food restrictions, as we discussed in the previous chapter, is not to say that we don't care about what we eat. Quite the contrary! Making all food permissible is how we eliminate food obsession that would otherwise lead to binging and weight gain. But it does not imply that meals become a free-for-all!

We want to be our own best friend and lifetime ally by striving to eat nutritiously every day to the best of our ability. Therefore, we purpose ourselves to eat an abundance of natural foods, such as vegetables, fruit, whole grains, nuts, legumes, protein, and fat from natural sources.

We *proactively* seek to avoid eating processed foods and food riddled with additives, preservatives, excessive sodium, white sugar, white flour, and processed oils (i.e., chemically-produced trans-fats, hydrogenated oils, etc.). Many such foods are associated with obesity, diabetes, hypertension, vascular disease, and other inflammatory diseases.

Time and time again I see patients lose weight *rapidly* and improve their health when processed food is reduced or eliminated from their diet and replaced with natural, whole foods.

Don't feel overwhelmed if this has not been your practice up until this point! ***What's important is that you start today!*** You are absolutely capable of doing this! Start with taking small, doable steps beginning with your very next meal.

For example, eat half the usual amount of your main course and replace the other half with fresh vegetables. Having pizza? Enjoy! Have *one* slice with a hefty salad, rather than 2 (or more) slices. Eat your sandwiches open faced with just one slice of bread, not two. Have a tall glass of water with every meal. Replace your usual dessert with a peach, nectarine, or some melon.

Not going for the fruit? Too much change too soon? That's fine. If chocolate's your thing, challenge yourself by eating just *half* the candy bar, or have just 2 cookies for dessert.

There are many possible nutritional improvements you can make at any meal. The idea is simply to ***do better at every meal than you have done previously so the outcome will be better than it has been previously.***

Start with whatever degree of improvement you are willing to make at your first meal, then your next. Your progress will be near automatic as you begin looking better and feeling *sensational!*

You will be *eager* to enhance your nutritional intake every chance you get because you will quickly experience the benefits! And you'll soon realize that the benefits of making these simple changes at each meal far outweigh the small, painless sacrifices.

This is how we become our own best friend and ally. By allowing *some* of what we love with *a lot* of what we need (if they are not one and the same). By performing small, healthy acts daily, we lose nothing (but weight and physical ailments) but gain everything!

Dieting depravation is replaced with meal satisfaction. Self-destructive behavior is replaced with acts of self-love and respect.

You will likely find that post-meal heaviness and sleepiness give way to increased energy and mental acuity. Chronic heartburn, bloating, and constipation may be replaced by improved digestion and bowel regulation.

Additionally, we don't need to count calories. But it's great to know that just by making healthier food choices as often as we can, we will naturally ingest fewer calories than we used to most days.

At each meal and snack, ask yourself how you can have the flavor of the food you desire while shaving off excess, unnecessary calories however you can. You won't miss eating them and you will lose weight effortlessly just by cutting them out.

Recall the egg salad sandwich I made on the first day of my NMD journey. Instead of thoughtlessly doing what I used to do (grabbing a pre-made sandwich made with whole eggs and 2 slices of bread, then adding extra, extra mayo), I thoughtfully and purposefully left out the extra, unneeded calories.

I used mainly egg whites (I kept one yolk), limited the mayo, and used only one slice of bread.

Making these simple changes did not diminish *the taste* **of my sandwich, but it shaved off over 300 calories that I would have otherwise eaten without giving it a second thought and with no added benefit!**

For dessert, I added fruit to my meal instead of the processed, prepackaged snack pack from the vending machine, thus sparing myself at least another 100 calories!

By being conscious about your meals and intentionally trimming off a mere 350 calories per day (not even *per meal* **as I did my first day), you could lose over 35 pounds in one year! This is significant because for most people, a 10 to 30-pound weight loss (5-10% of one's body weight) can reduce diabetes, hypertension, inflammation, the risk of heart disease and stroke, sleep apnea, and obesity-related infertility.**

I once met a woman who lost 30 pounds within 3 months just by swapping full-calorie drinks for non-caloric drinks and by cutting off her day's eating by 6:00 pm. She did absolutely nothing else! These 2 minor changes produced major results!

Many of you have had 30 pounds you've wanted to lose for years. But you've been waiting to muster up enough willpower to diet (aka: be hungry, miserable, and eat food you hate for a long, long time). Not surprisingly the day of muster never came. Or it came, you dieted, lost the weight, took one bite of food you love, and were unable to stop eating until all your weight was regained.

This is because *the restriction of dieting is not sustainable* and sustainability is critical for us who struggle (or *have* struggled, like myself) with obesity and compulsive eating.

Furthermore, as we discussed in the previous chapter, the restriction of dieting leads to overeating/binging. The pendulum swings *from all to nothing and back again* when we approach weight loss from this *diet mentality*.

Simply making a conscious effort to increase healthy food on our plate, while decreasing less-healthy food, and by avoiding unnecessary calories, is clearly an easier, more effective, *sustainable* approach to weight loss and weight maintenance than is dieting.

A word to the wise in closing this chapter: While practicing new skills and developing new habits, don't expect to be perfect! You may revert to old behaviors at times. But don't panic! Do not think that you *can't* do this. You can!

Be patient and encourage yourself as you would a child learning to walk. You may take a few steps forward and then fall down, but this is par for the course. Your fall-frequency will decrease as you discover what works best for you and as you settle into your own unique rhythm.

Notice I said that *falls decrease* rather than saying they *stop*. Indeed, I still fall periodically. I'm not superhuman, but rather an ongoing work in progress. I'm totally fine with this.

As long as we are human, chances are that we will still fall now and again. What matters is that we immediately get back up and resume our NMD lifestyle.

I'll humbly share about one of my recent falls in the chapter *Don't Expect Perfection. Just Do Your Best Each Day!* I'll also explain what I do when I fall to immediately recover so that when I slip-up it's no big deal.

Summary of NMD Principle #2
Always Strive to Make Healthy Choices

We proactively strive to make healthier choices every day, meal by meal, beginning with the very next meal.

WHEN SHOULD I EAT?

MIND

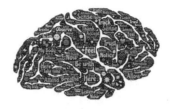

EAT WHENEVER YOU ARE TRULY HUNGRY

NMD MINDSET PRINCIPLE #3

*H*unger is our body's way of telling us to provide the fuel it needs to perform its daily functions. While the chronic dieter tries *not* to eat, NMD on the other hand teaches us to eat whenever we are truly hungry. This is a natural and healthy response to our body's call for food.

Aside from purposeful fasting, going without food and fluids for extended periods can cause immediate and chronic health problems, including low blood sugar, low blood pressure, dehydration, electrolyte imbalance, and more.

Additionally, the body responds to prolonged periods without eating by slowing down metabolism and *holding on to fat* in order to prepare and survive for potential famine. Slowing down metabolism makes it harder to lose weight at that time and in the future. This is obviously the exact opposite of what the dieter intended.

Furthermore, going hungry for extended periods usually back-fires and results in binging, ultimately leading to weight gain rather than loss. It's actually healthier to remain at the same weight (even if one is obese) than it is to 'yo-yo' diet with repeated weight losses and gains.

Thus, we see that the dieter's mindset of trying *not to eat* when truly hungry is unhealthy, counterproductive, and futile. ***It is normal and healthy to eat when our bodies call for food.***

So when your stomach is growling, or you feel an emptiness or a gnawing in your gut, it's time to eat. If you don't feel these particular signs but are feeling lightheaded or mildly dizzy, ask yourself how long it has been since you last had a meal or drank fluids. If it has been several hours, these may signs that you've gone too long without eating or hydrating, and it's now time to nourish your body.

~

Summary of NMD Principle #3
Eat Whenever You Are Truly Hungry

We practice recognizing our body's physiologic cues that indicate true hunger. We respond by eating. No starving allowed!

STOP EATING AS SOON AS YOUR BODY (NOT YOUR TASTE BUDS OR EMOTIONAL STATE) IS SATISFIED

NMD MINDSET PRINCIPLE #4

*W*e have discussed eating when we are authentically hungry, as indicated by our body's physiologic cues. Our next step is to *practice recognizing the cues of physiologic satisfaction* when we are eating and to grow in the discipline of ending our meal at that point.

During the course of our day, we find ourselves eating meals and snacks on the go, in the car, during meetings, in front of the TV and the computer. But despite all of the distractions, when we eat we must practice paying attention to the signals our body sends when it is satisfied and requires no additional food.

Such indicators include the *absence* of hunger, a sense of pressure or fullness in the gut, and a decreased sense of taste. These signs are produced as a result of complex signaling that involves neurotransmitters and hormones of the nervous system and the gastrointestinal system respectively.

This is the means by which our bodies communicate the message to us that it has received sufficient nutrition and we need not eat any further. We gain weight when we eat beyond our body's needs so this is a habit that we must break.

In practicing awareness of your body's cues, notice that after a while when eating a meal, the food no longer excites your taste buds like it did when you took your first few bites. The explosive celebration in your mouth fizzles out. Soon, every bite starts tasting the same.

Your taste buds are now barely firing. You also feel some pressure in your belly and the hunger you had when you began eating is gone. The party's over. Your body is satisfied so it's time to stop eating.

You're amazed (and may want to curse) when you realize how little food it actually took to fill your stomach and satisfy your body. You may discover that you have been in the habit of eating twice as much food than you actually need. But don't fret when it's time to stop eating.

I know how delicious it is and how fun it is to eat it, but you don't have to overeat. You can literally continue eating the same food the very next time you are hungry. That's just a few hours away (more or less) so I know you're able to wait!

Wrap the remaining food up in cellophane, put it in the fridge, and move on with your day. It's really that simple. You can finish it at your next meal if you want.

Don't feel guilty at times if you eat beyond your body's signals (whether deliberately or unconsciously). The more we eat at any one time, the longer it takes to get hungry again. So if you went a little overboard but *immediately resumed adhering to your body's cues* by not eating again until the next time you were hungry, you should be fine. Be sure to stop eating at the earliest sign of satisfaction at your next meal.

Our bodies have a way of compensating to maintain equilibrium when we veer off course. For a period of time after overeating, we'll get hungry less frequently and become satisfied a little sooner when we eat.

Ingesting less calories during this time will off-set the extra calories we ingested when we overate. All will balance out if we simply resume living the NMD principles.

When we overeat, it's critical to NOT backslide into practicing the *diet mentality* of saying to ourselves, "Well, I really blew it! I might as well *go all the way*. I'll get back on track tomorrow." Which actually means you've given yourself permission to binge. NO! Please abandon this way of thinking!

We no longer *plan* to overeat just because we haven't been 'perfect' in our eating. Overeating here and there does NOT make or keep us fat (skinny people overeat too by the way). It's the extreme *all or nothing, perfection or destruction* way of thinking that does!

Perfectionism is a set-up for failure (discussed further *in the chapter Don't Expect Perfection. Just Do Your Best Each Day!*) so we don't practice it within the NMD lifestyle. It's cruel and unrealistic to expect perfection every time we eat (which is, give or take about 100 times per month!).

Ironically, we make far more progress in losing weight and improving our health when we loosen up a little rather than being so rigid.

The goal is to **do your best each day** to respect the cues your body sends you. Eat when it signals to eat. Stop eating when it signals to stop. Don't eat again until it signals to eat again (**discussed in the following chapter *Don't Eat Again Until You're Truly Hungry***).

When (not *if*) you deviate off course, simply resume the above ASAP. Commit to this and to the other NMD principles, and you'll lose weight peaceably and almost effortlessly.

Summary of NMD Principle #4
Stop Eating Once Your Body is Satisfied

When eating, we practice recognizing our body's physiologic cues that indicate satisfaction (*satiation*) and fullness (*satiety*). We respond by ending our meals at that point.

DON'T EAT AGAIN UNTIL YOU'RE TRULY HUNGRY

NMD MINDSET PRINCIPLE #5

Once we have finished eating a meal, we don't eat again until the next time we're truly hungry. This means no random snacking between meals or comfort eating to relieve anxiety, depression, anger, loneliness, or other emotional and psychological states.

Work on breaking the habit of continuous munching in front of the TV or at the movies if your body is not signaling to eat. Learn to say "No thank you." in social settings when you're offered food if you're not authentically hungry.

Because temptations arise from every corner of our lives, from TV commercials, to billboards, to social events, and so on, we have the opportunity to grow in discipline rapidly as we practice abstaining from impulsively and compulsively eating throughout each day.

Each time we exercise self-control and decline to eat when we're not truly hungry, we get stronger and saying "No thank you." gets easier. Soon the habit of *not eating outside of true hunger* becomes second nature.

～

Most of us know people who have severe food allergies. When the food they are allergic to is set before them, they immediately reject it without hesitation. They've had years of experience in saying "No thank you." to these foods, so their resolve to avoid it is solid. They know the price they'll pay if they were to indulge and they determined long ago that it's just not worth it.

And so should our mindset be with respect to eating impulsively. The price we pay (obesity) is just not worth it. So we strive not to eat unless we're *authentically* hungry.

～

Summary of NMD Principle #5
Don't Eat Again Until You're Truly Hungry

We practice not eating outside of true hunger.

WHAT IS MY MINDSET?

MIND

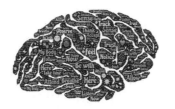

DON'T EXPECT PERFECTION. JUST DO YOUR BEST EACH DAY!

NMD MINDSET PRINCIPLE #6

*I*n living the NMD lifestyle, *our daily goal is to do our best* to eat and live according to the principles and to take action steps daily. We purpose ourselves to grow and progress consistently in all of these areas. But we do not expect perfection.

Many compulsive behaviors and addictions have clear and distinct points of sobriety and abstinence. Alcoholics are sober when they no longer drink and smokers are abstinent when they no longer smoke.

But the lines are blurred for the compulsive eater because we can't give up our *drug of choice* (food!). Not just daily, but multiple times a day, for the remainder of our lives, we have to consume this tempting 'substance' without allowing ourselves to be consumed *by it*.

With several choices to make regarding food and eating every single day, it's unrealistic to think that we're going to get it right each time. To expect perfection is unreasonable and is a set-up for failure. But we can, and indeed should commit to putting forth our best efforts to live within the NMD principles every day.

By consistently *doing our personal best* (which will vary day by day, sometimes even hour by hour), we will indeed lose weight and gain freedom from compulsive eating.

When (*not if*) you veer off course and overeat (or even completely lose it and binge), do not get discouraged and don't overreact. Simply assess the situation and determine how you can do better next time. Immediately carry on with the NMD mindset principles and action steps.

Wait to eat again until you are authentically hungry and eat only the amount of food your body needs to be satisfied. Make the healthiest meals possible, starting with your very next meal.

Whatever you do, do not *panic and go back into the bondage of dieting!* That would be the worst thing you could do! **You must walk through the learning process of living a diet-free life.** This includes learning from your mistakes. Like a toddler learning to walk, you're going to fall sometimes. That's a given.

But the next time you're tempted to go off course, you'll be more experienced and better equipped to handle the situation. This is the process, there's no way around it.

To be honest, I still veer off my dietary trajectory at times. For instance, I once went on vacation with friends during the week of Thanksgiving (double temptation!). My friend Ava who's an amazing cook was hosting.

Aside from the phenomenal spread we knew to expect on Thanksgiving, Ava prepared a different homemade feast just about every day. What's a weight loss doctor to do? Ava's home cooking is just not to be missed! I had to balance *indulgence* with *discipline and grace*.

I purposed myself to stick to the NMD principals and action steps to the best of my ability. I was successful in waiting until I was hungry to eat **(MIND Principle #5)**.

I didn't eat outside of true hunger throughout the week. This meant I wasn't feasting at every opportunity that presented itself. That wasn't a problem. I'd make a plate of edible goodness and save it for later when I would get hungry.

I also continued prioritizing my health **(Action Step #1)**. I had brought my blender with me and made green drinks every day **(Action Step #4)**. I also exercised more days than not **(Action Step #2)**.

What I struggled with most was putting the fork down when my body was satisfied at each and every smorgasbord! I confess that I didn't execute this NMD principle **(MIND Principle #4)** perfectly. Fortunately, I know the futility of expecting perfection from *imperfect me*, so I didn't sweat it too much when I missed the mark.

With the *prolonged absence of hunger* that followed each of my indulgences, I usually wasn't hungry for the remainder of the day. So I would just pass on the next buffet meal that was offered **(MIND Principle #5)**.

Of course, I had to face the day of reckoning. There was no avoiding it. Upon returning home, I got on the scale. I was 4 pounds heavier. Awesome! Totally worth it! But I clearly needed to do a little 'damage repair.'

Did I do anything *radical* to take the extra weight off? No way! My NMD lifestyle remained the same as it had been for years, but I ran a tighter ship. I was proactive in my efforts to do my very best, but I didn't deviate from my usual regimen.

For instance, I was less apt to allow my schedule to interfere with my exercise routine and I was careful to stop eating when my body suggested to do so (no prolonged fork activity). The weight naturally came off as a result.

Two weeks later my weight was the same as it was before I went on vacation. This process was virtually effortless and it was definitely stress-free! This is why I'm ok with living imperfectly - as long as I live responsibly. This means after loosening the reigns and having some fun, I tighten them back up for a while. *But I don't go to one extreme or another.*

My weight may teeter-totter sometimes, but it always balances out. For the most part, I've maintained my 50+ pound weight loss for about 8 years as of the writing of this book.

~

Vacations, holidays, parties, and celebrations are all part of the fruit of life, and we should enjoy them thoroughly (in a moderate, not destructive way). When (not *if*) you act up a little, don't sweat it! Just:

#1: Make sure the food is worth it (like on the level of Ava's morsels!).

#2: Don't beat yourself up in the aftermath.

#3: Resume your NMD lifestyle ASAP! Tighten the reigns if need be. You'll see your weight begin dropping again.

~

Summary of NMD Principle #6
Don't Expect Perfection. Just Do Your Best Each Day!

In NMD, we don't expect perfection (that's a set-up for failure) nor do we purposely *'throw in the towel'* and pig-out just because we slipped up. Instead, we do our best to live by the NMD principles and to take action steps every day. We strive to practice moderation at all times.

When we veer off course in any way, we don't beat ourselves up, give up, or revert back to old, destructive habits. We simply reflect on how to do better in the future and we immediately resume our NMD lifestyle (+/- some damage repair).

No extremes. No perfection. No stress.

START TODAY. ALWAYS TODAY!

NMD MINDSET PRINCIPLE #7

*T*he wisdom of ancient text says ***be transformed by the renewing of your mind***.

Indeed, all that we say, do, and think contributes to shaping our beliefs and attitudes. By taking immediate action, you begin establishing a mindset that is characterized by achieving, accomplishing, succeeding, and winning.

Mindset Principle #7 is all about taking action and living your dreams *today* rather than *someday*. You will begin today developing invaluable habits and breaking old, destructive ones.

Commit to practicing the NMD principles when you eat your very next meal. Take at least one action step today as well.

No preparation is needed to get started. No products need to be purchased, no money needs to be spent. You can practice any or all of the NMD principles and action steps just by deciding to do so!

Write down the steps you plan to take and check them off each time you accomplish one. If you don't end up accomplishing all of them today, that's fine! Don't fret! Just try again tomorrow.

Remember, perfection is never the goal (it doesn't exist anyway). Doing your daily best and being consistent is what counts!

There's no need to be overwhelmed. The NMD lifestyle is entirely doable because each person begins and progresses at their own pace and according to their own ability. It doesn't matter if you start by taking great leaps or small steps. I happen to be a baby-stepper myself. *Inch by inch, life is a cinch; yard by yard, life can be hard!*

Life demands we live it *yard by yard* at times, but when I have liberty, I prefer the *inch* approach. This is not to say I want to take forever to reach my goals. It's to say I want to *ensure* that I reach my goals. Anybody can start the race strong, but most will poop-out, and few will finish.

Slow and steady **wins the race. Because slow and steady is sustainable.**

By taking consistent, bite-sized steps over time, I'm thankful to have been able to reconstruct my entire life and to design the life I always dreamt of having.

And it all begun by taking the first step.

So start today. *Always* today!

Summary of NMD Principle #7
Start Today. *Always* Today!

Start living your NMD lifestyle *today! Now!* Practice the MIND principles beginning with your next meal. Take an action step or two from MOTION. If you stumble and fall, don't worry! Just get back on track and resume your NMD lifestyle ASAP.

Always strive to take action the very same day!

TESTIMONIAL ~ IMPERFECTLY PERFECT!

SHANNON'S STORY

*S*hannon was a registered nurse in her 40s. She was a mom of grown kids and worked the night shift at a local hospital. She led a sedentary lifestyle and had been obese for most of her life. So she approached me for obesity treatment.

I counseled Shannon on the NMD lifestyle, but she was skeptical that she could lose weight by *letting go* of all the rules and regulations that accompany diets. This was the opposite of all she had tried (and failed) her whole life. But she had struggled with her weight for so long that she was willing to give it a try.

While obtaining her dietary history, Shannon sheepishly confided in me that every morning after working the night shift, she was in the habit of eating a very large meal without any restrictions.

This was her '*me time*.' It was enjoyable and relaxing, and she was forthright in letting me know she had no intention of giving this practice up any time soon. I get it.

Like heading to the bar each day after work, a daily mini-binge was Shannon's way of unwinding. Been there. This was no time to wag a finger in judgment. That was the last thing Shannon needed. Like most compulsive eaters, if she could do better, she would do better.

I convinced Shannon that it was okay to start right from where she was at that time (where else *could* she start from?), as long as she was willing to begin taking steps towards improving her lifestyle right away.

So I asked her directly if she would be willing to *do her best* to stop eating once her body signals that she's had enough to eat **(NMD Principle #4)** and to work on improving the *quality* of her meals on a regular basis **(NMD Principle #2)** along with practicing the other NMD Principles.

She said she was willing but wasn't shy to let me know that she doubted she could lose weight *just by trying*. Fair enough. I realize that the NMD mindset is counterintuitive for most. So all I require of my patients is a willingness to do their daily best. The proof of the method is in the results.

I then pursued a commitment to get active.

Shannon had not exercised in years and she was not in good condition. She would get short of breath walking up stairs and walking moderate distances, like across a parking lot. I asked Shannon if she would work on increasing her fitness by being active to some degree on a daily basis.

This could be as simple as putting on tennis shoes and going for short walks at whatever pace she was able and for as long as she was able. There was no pressure to exercise longer or with more intensity than she was able to do. The duration and intensity of her exercise would naturally increase as long as she was consistently active.

As with all patients, I counseled Shannon to begin right away by taking baby steps from her authentic starting place. I asked that she commit to doing her best to improve and advance her efforts in living her NMD lifestyle every day *as she was able*. Perfection was not required.

With 100% certainty, I knew she would lose weight with daily applied effort. As her weight began going down, her confidence and motivation would rise, as would her energy and sense of wellbeing.

Her improved mental and physical health would enable her to apply even more effort toward her NMD lifestyle, which in turn would enhance her weight loss. And so the cycle of positive reinforcement goes.

Shannon agreed to all of the above. She recognized that her biggest challenge would likely be trying to stop eating once her body has enough, at least during her first meal after working the night shift. So she purposed herself to apply concentrated effort in that one particular area.

She appreciated however that there were no foods that were *off-limits*, so her favorite meal of the day was still satisfying. As promised, Shannon incorporated exercise into her daily life.

She started by just walking on the treadmill ten minutes a day at a comfortable pace.

I followed up with Shannon weekly. She was surprised and delighted by the ease of her new lifestyle. She was eating less and a bit healthier in the morning, and she was slowly but surely tolerating more exercise.

She perceived her clothes fitting looser, but she refused to weigh herself. She was so afraid of being disappointed after daring to hope (again) that she had really found a way to lose weight. But finally her curiosity was greater than she could resist, so she got on the scale.

She was shocked and thrilled to see that she had lost 17 pounds in three weeks! She was so encouraged because she was living in a way that she was able to sustain.

The NMD lifestyle didn't require her to do more than she was capable of at any time. She simply had to *do her best daily* from the sincere place wherein she stood at any given time. No more was expected of her and no less.

Shannon and I were both ecstatic at her progress!

MOTION

TAKING ACTION!
GETTING INTO MOTION!

MOTION

INTRODUCTION

Excellence is not a singular act, but a habit.
We are what we repeatedly do. ~ **Aristotle**

Permanent change begins with our thoughts and beliefs, so we first discussed adopting the 7 NMD Mindset Principles. But, a healthy mindset must be accompanied by *action* in order to be profitable and produce change.

Haven't you heard that *faith without works is dead?*

~

There are 4 Action Steps that make up the *MOTION* component of No More Dieting. Each step is listed below followed by a detailed discussion.

- Action Step #1: Make Health Your Top Priority!
- Action Step #2: Move That Body!
- Action Step #3: Accountability and Support
- Action Step #4: Seven Simple Steps to Live an Energized Life. *When We Feel Better, We Do Better!*

MAKE HEALTH YOUR TOP PRIORITY!

*U*ndoubtedly, our body is our greatest possession. A masterpiece in which we live that allows us to do literally *all* that we do. Nothing at all can be done by a human unless it is first initiated through their body.

When a body no longer functions, nothing more can be accomplished by its occupant. Therefore, it's imperative that we optimize and maintain the function of this miraculous machine through which all possibilities occur. Yet we don't.

We invest a vast amount of time and money in obtaining and maintaining our cherished computers, appliances, vehicles, and dwellings. But remarkably, relatively little is invested in the system that allows for use and enjoyment of these things.

We also invest time, money, and energy into the lives of our loved ones, yet not into the instrument through which our love is expressed and received.

We know all of this, but don't care to consider it. It's the kind of truth we typically reflect on when we, or someone we know, is gravely ill. Prior to that, there's always an excuse to neglect our body.

I don't have time to exercise **we say.**

But when health is poor and we get sick, precious time slips away with doctors appointments or while home in bed. Quality time with our family is lost as is time being productive in business.

I can't afford healthy food **we proclaim.**

But hospital bills, insurance copays, and prescription medicine for chronic conditions are far more costly. And if we're honest, we'd admit to squandering time and money on things *far* less important than our health.

How much time do we waste on the internet, phone, and TV? How much money is blown on fast food, junk food, restaurants, coffee houses, juice bars, entertainment, unnecessary gadgets, and attire?

They're all pleasurable, I agree. But if we're splurging on these things while making excuses for neglecting our health, we're living in denial and gambling with our very lives!

We can't afford to take our bodies for granted any longer. The risk is too great. We have to make our health top priority!

If it means withdrawing time and money from less important activities and redistributing them in support of our weight loss goals, so be it. This is not a selfish act.

On the contrary, to *not* address our weight is to risk depriving others of the best and the most we have to give. Moreover, obesity-related illness can lead to incapacitation and even death. This obviously burdens the hearts and lives of others.

Putting our health first is not only an act of self-love, but it is the most responsible thing we can do for all involved.

As with any serious goal, intentional weight loss and healthy living require forethought and commitment. Time must be allotted for meal-planning, shopping, cooking, and exercise.

I understand all too well how challenging it is to squeeze time out of a schedule where it appears none exists. But I can attest to the fact that *it can be done* if we want success bad enough!

Summary of NMD Action Step #1
Make Health Your Top Priority!

Our ability to live life to the fullest is directly proportional to our state of health. So, what could be more important than keeping the vehicle through which live, tuned up and running properly?

We must make health our top priority!

MOVE THAT BODY!

ACTION STEP #2

*T*he benefits of exercise cannot be overstated. Moderate exercise is associated with a reduction in *all-cause mortality.* This means that the rate of death (no matter what the cause) is reduced in the population of people who exercise.

Exercise also reduces the risk of type 2 diabetes, high blood pressure, and vascular disease including heart attacks, stroke, kidney disease, and the list goes on. When these conditions are already present, exercise can reduce their severity and help to prevent recurrence.

Additionally, exercise reduces depression, anxiety, and helps with stress management. So adopting it as a part of our healthy lifestyle is vital.

Unfortunately, many people consider exercise laborious, so they struggle with the notion of making it a part of their daily routine.

But exercise need not be synonymous with 'work.' The key is to make it fun! Choose to do activities that you truly enjoy. If you've wasted money in the past on unused gym memberships, going to the gym is probably not for you. So think outside the box.

How about trying a home workout program? There are countless options via DVD, cable, and the internet. There are free yoga, pilates, and step classes on YouTube. If you're an outdoors person, try walking, hiking, skating, biking, swimming, or investing in a backyard trampoline.

Maybe there's a certain type of dance you've been wanting to learn, like African, Zumba, salsa, tap, ballroom, hip hop, or pole dancing. Get creative! I'll be honest and admit that I like to jam around the kitchen while cooking dinner, despite my kids' embarrassment. I can hear them now, "Oh boy! Mommy's getting her groove on again." Eyes rolling.

The possibilities are endless!

How about joining a family sports team at your local recreational center? Maybe a basketball, softball, or soccer team? Consider family walks or short bike rides after dinner. Or, if you're committed to watching TV after work, maybe put a treadmill, elliptical, or stationary bike in front of your big screen (my husband did this).

If you already have a machine, take the clothes off of it and hang them up in the closet where they belong, dust it off, hop on, and get moving!

I ask my patients to recall activities they used to enjoy way back in the day before life became too busy. Most can readily come up with an activity or two that they would love to do again if they had time.

I remind them that we all have 24 hours a day and our health must be our first priority (**see the chapter *Make Health Your Top Priority!*)**. Then I ask that they begin doing some form of activity right away, even if it's just to walk around the block for starters.

Few people will maintain a course of exercise they find too physically strenuous or mentally overwhelming. So I advise patients to choose whatever activity they like and start at whatever level of intensity and duration they are comfortable with doing.

Encouraging patients (and you!) to start at their own comfort level is essential in helping them to become immediately active. And as with all NMD principles and action steps, our next goal is to proactively strive to make improvements every day, even if they seem small.

My sister Jaimie told me that when she started exercising after years of living a sedentary lifestyle, she began with only doing five minutes a day on her stationary bike. She would get so winded, she couldn't tolerate more than that when she first began.

But every few days, she would add a few more minutes to her regimen and found that she could cycle with more intensity. Now she enjoys high-intensity aerobic classes that she streams from the internet into her living room just about every day.

This underscores the point that it's more important to *just get started* with the NMD principles and action steps, and improve daily as you are able than it is to try to aim for some imagined *perfection*. More often than not, perfectionism leads to quitting, so modest beginnings with regular improvement over time is always preferred. This approach is more physically and psychologically sustainable, so we are more likely to adopt an active lifestyle and maintain it for life, and that's the goal!

'Modest' exercise is different for each person. It may be 10 minutes of walking for one, 30 minutes of swimming for another, or 60 minutes of kitchen-grooving for someone else.

Consult your physician before starting an exercise regimen, and begin at your unique point of ability.

Summary of NMD Action Step #2
Move That Body!

Consistent exercise reduces the risk of numerous diseases and increases our health and quality of life. So, adopting it as part of our NMD lifestyle is one way we prioritize our health.

The key to embracing exercise is to make it your playtime! Discover fun activities, so exercise won't feel like work, but rather a *reprieve* from work.

ACCOUNTABILITY AND SUPPORT

ACTION STEP #3

*H*aving support can help lighten the load when we are working toward our weight loss goals and accountability can help to keep us on track.

Many people find it helpful to utilize a friend or family member as their means of support. This can be as simple as checking in via phone, text, or email to declare your daily goals in the morning and to confirm that they've been accomplished each night.

You could report your daily or weekly weight if that motivates you to stay on track. If you prefer anonymity, an online forum might be your best choice for accountability and camaraderie.

For exercise accountability, try having a walking or jogging buddy, or join a biking or hiking group. There are meet-up groups online where you can look for groups of people in your area who share your interests and meet regularly to do them together.

There are lots of websites, mobile apps, and electronic devices to help keep you accountable. Some keep track of your physical activity, and caloric, carbohydrate, fat, protein, and water intake. There are numerous options to choose from!

Whether you prefer electronics or more of a human touch, being accountable and utilizing support can help you stay focused on your goals and keep you on track. Explore different resources until you find the people and tools that are best suited for you.

~

Summary of NMD Action Step #3
Accountability and Support

Like a leaf in the breeze, support can be uplifting; bearing us up through rain or shine. Accountability helps to keep us on track when we're weary and tempted to slack.

Seek out a supportive accountability partner. This can help ensure that you reach your goals while adding joy to the journey along the way.

SEVEN SIMPLE STEPS TO LIVING AN ENERGIZED LIFE!

ACTION STEP #4

When We Feel Better, We Do Better!

*a*s I mentioned elsewhere, losing weight is just the tip of the iceberg! Once we shift our mindset and take action consistently (no matter how big or small), we will be rewarded with consistent results. Learning this skillset is the gift that keeps on giving because this same process can be applied to reach any goal!

However, it's difficult to accomplish much of anything when we feel fatigue and lethargic. We must be *energized* if we are to live the high quality, purposeful lives we were born to live!

This chapter provides 7 tips to help turbocharge your No More Dieting lifestyle!

1. Nutritional Supplementation: What Does the Science Say?

The increasing prevalence of diet-related vitamin and mineral deficiencies in our society is undeniable, as is the medical conditions associated with them.

Although a healthy diet is the ideal source for essential vitamins and minerals, the rising rate of deficiencies indicate that our current diets are grossly falling short.

Fortunately, scientific studies show that diet-related deficiencies can be corrected largely by taking the appropriate nutritional supplements. It behooves us therefore not only to improve the quality of our food intake but to consider adding quality nutritional supplements to our health regimen when and if appropriate.

In today's health and nutrition market you can find anything from standard, OTC supplements, to pharmaceutical-grade, customized supplements.

Check with your physician before taking any supplements and/or beginning a new dietary regimen.

2. Green Drinks

I started making green drinks (fruit and vegetable smoothies) when my youngest son Daniel was a toddler because he stubbornly refused to eat just about all fruits and most vegetables.

Out of desperation, I threw his veggies in a blender, added some apple and frozen banana, and served it to him with a straw (*Eureka! He drank it!*). Eventually, I began serving green drinks to my entire family as a fast and easy way of ensuring we all got a hardy dose of vitamins, minerals, and fiber every day.

I passed the baton to my oldest son, Joshua when he was 10 by teaching him how to make the family's green drinks. From that point on, he's provided us with this health-supporting, liquid energy on a daily basis (thank you, Lovie!).

Green drinks have become such an important part of our family's health routine that we hardly go a day without them. When I miss a day of having my drink, there's a notable decrease in my energy, mental acuity, and my work efficiency.

My mood is not as great on these days either, and I tend to get tired sooner. This puts my family at higher risk of the *Momster* coming out as the day wears on (as Josh refers to me when I'm tired and cranky).

Certainly *eating* a hearty amount of raw fruits and vegetables every day would produce the same energy and health-support, but blending has its unique advantages.

When blending, we can mix just about any combination of fruits, vegetables, and healthy supplements to get a wide variety of nutrients all in one glass.

It's also great when time is limited because blending is so efficient. *Just blend, pour, and take 'em out the door!* (corny perhaps, but isn't it catchy?...just a little?). It beats grabbing a pastry, some fast food, or skipping a meal altogether when we're on the go.

You may also find that your caloric intake is less on the days that you 'drink' your salad. I, for instance, *adore* white, creamy salad dressing (not the low-fat stuff either) and wouldn't consider eating a salad without it. I also butter my cooked vegetables shamelessly.

When I drink instead of eat my veggies, I'm sparing my body hundreds of calories in salad dressing or butter that I would have otherwise ingested. This translates to fewer pounds on my body over time.

I should touch on the difference between juicing and blending. With juicing, the voluminous fiber is strained out and only juice is extracted. With blending, the entire fruit and vegetable are used, so all of the fiber is retained.

Ounce for ounce, juicing requires a *much* higher quantity of fruits and vegetables to produce the same volume of juice compared to blending. Because of the quantity of produce needed for daily juicing, it can be a challenging regimen to maintain in terms of cost, shopping frequency, and storage space in the refrigerator. But, the benefit of juicing is that the juice is more concentrated in nutrients compared to the juice of blending.

The benefits of fiber, which you get with blending, include weight loss, improved cholesterol, a lower risk of heart disease and cancer, and improved intestinal health. I happen to blend, but many people prefer juicing. You can't go wrong with either practice.

My family's basic blend includes the following superfoods:

Kale, spinach, various berries, some apple, carrots, tomatoes, cucumbers, and frozen banana. Other high-energy foods to blend include other leafy greens (e.g. mustard or collard), bell peppers, broccoli, beets, ginger, garlic, and herbs. Some people add flax, chia seed, wheatgrass, and yogurt. The healthy options are endless!

To avoid unnecessary calories and concentrated sugar, we blend using water as the base liquid, rather than fruit juice. The apple and banana provide adequate sweetness. If you decide to blend and want to use bananas, wait until they are maximally ripe (with brown spots) before removing the peel. Once the peel is removed, slice them up and put them in a freezer bag, and freeze them.

Frozen bananas provide a thick, frothiness that gives blended drinks the consistency and sweetness of a smoothie or shake. Add to taste. I use only a few slices while my kids use about half a banana.

We also add 'super green' and 'super red' powders to our green drinks. These are antioxidant-rich supplements that are comprised of vegetables, fruit, spirulina, chlorella, probiotics, and more. You can find them online or at your local health food store.

I urge you to commit to at least one week of making and drinking green drinks every day if you're not in the habit of doing so already. Consider having one for breakfast with some protein, or maybe have it as a meal replacement.

Once you experience the energy, mental sharpness, and sense of wellness that comes from drinking green drinks on a daily basis, you'll never want to go a day without one!

3. Shakes as Snacks and Meal Replacements

Eating and drinking natural, whole foods is always preferred over processed foods. But realistically, there are times when our schedules interfere with shopping or food preparation. There are also times we find ourselves in a situation where food options are limited or grossly unhealthy.

And there are yet other times when, doggone it, we just want a shake! It's during such times when meal replacement shakes can come in handy.

There are a wide variety of shakes and meal replacement products on the market these days. High protein, low carb, organic, gluten-free, vegan, kosher, you name it! There's something for everyone. You may benefit from finding shakes you like and keeping them stored at work and at home.

Alternatively, you may enjoy making fresh, homemade shakes to take with you to work. My family enjoys a simple blend of unsweetened almond milk or coconut milk with flavored stevia drops. My kids especially love chocolate-flavored stevia drops stirred in milk as a dessert (chocolate milk! Ta-da!). I often will have a glass on the run or at my desk with a hard-boiled egg or two. A fast, convenient, yet filling meal!

Although not a true shake, just having some milk with a squirt of stevia for flavor (or for sweetness if you're having plant-based, unsweetened milk) might be just the thing to keep hunger at bay in a pinch. No blending required for this quickie. Just stir. For a more fully-balanced meal add berries, banana, some protein powder, and blend.

Having a shake close by to tide you over when you're hungry might be the very thing that rescues you from giving in and eating something you'll later regret. And the portability of shakes makes them convenient enough to keep stocked.

If you have metabolic disorders (e.g. type 1 or type 2 diabetes, metabolic syndrome, etc.) or other chronic disorders, you must consider which products are most appropriate for you given your particular medical status.

As always, consult with your physician before adopting any new dietary practices.

4. Hydrate for Health *and Weight Loss!*

Water is vital to the life and function of every cell in our body. It makes up about 60-70% of our body's volume (more in infants), so it's easy to see why maintaining adequate hydration is of primary importance.

One of the ways our bodies regulate fluid volume is by means of the hypothalamus, which is located in the brain. Of its many duties, as a 'thirst center' it recognizes when we're in need of more water. It then sends out a signal of *thirst*.

But many of us miss the memo. Misinterpreting the signal, we may respond inappropriately. Or underestimating the importance, we just ignore our thirst altogether. But we pay for it dearly with fatigue, malaise, achiness, dry lips, dry mouth, and possibly worse, depending on how fluid depleted we are and our body's ability to compensate.

The hypothalamus is also responsible for sending signals that regulate hunger and satiety (the sense of fullness we get when eating). So it's possible to misinterpret thirst for hunger and to eat when our body is actually signaling for water.

To avoid the risk of dehydration (and unnecessary caloric intake), proactively strive to drink an adequate amount of fluid each day. The standard recommendation is to drink at least 2 liters (8 cups) per day, but due to varying age and medical conditions, the amount will be different for some.

Check with your doctor regarding the appropriate amount of fluid intake for you.

I recommend drinking as much of your fluids in the form of pure water as you can. But if you're like my husband and insist on 'flavoring' your water, don't use the chemical-laden, artificially-flavored powder packets. Shoot for natural options.

5. Sleep is Essential!

At least 7 hours of sleep each night is recommended for optimal health. Not getting enough sleep works against us in several ways.

There are negative, hormonally-induced effects that include increased hunger and a decreased sense of fullness, both of which can contribute to overeating when we're tired.

Preservation of stored fat also occurs when we don't get enough sleep (God forbid!).

Also, when we're mentally and physically sluggish, we're less apt to grocery shop or prepare healthy meals. We're at higher risk of yielding to rising cravings for comfort food, such as sugary, starchy, and fried foods.

These may lend a brief pick-me-up, but we know the crash is soon coming. We are also not likely to maintain a regular exercise regimen if we're chronically tired or fatigued.

If you're getting less than 7 hours of sleep per night and are experiencing some of the effects noted above, it's imperative to your weight loss and overall health that you increase your sleep time.

Just by adding an extra hour or two each night, you may notice an increase of mood and energy, as well as improved eating behavior and the desire to eat higher-quality foods.

6. Dress It, Don't Neglect It!

Reflecting self-love and respect in our dress has a powerful impact on our thoughts, which affects all else, including our energy and behavior.

Consider the energy that radiates from us when we look our best. We walk and talk with more confidence, we're more productive at work, we even tend to eat less at meals. Compare this to the energy we emit when we're in the 'ol baggy sweats and tee-shirt. I won't even go there.

Why the difference in energy? *We adopt the characteristics of the garments we wear.* Our dress also influences how we're treated by others.

When we neglect our appearance due to our size, we're giving credence to the false, yet prevalent notion that a person's value is based on physical attributes. How sad!

On the contrary, you are a miracle! Size has no bearing on that. So do away with the frumpy attire. Dress *today* how you imagine yourself dressing when you reach your goal weight.

Don't wait until you lose weight to sport a nice suit, a gorgeous dress, or the cute jeans that you've admired from afar. You are no less worthy of adorning yourself *today!*

To be clear, the point is not to 'dress-up' per se. There's nothing *inherently* wrong with sweats and tees, or any other casual, comfortable wear (I'm in scrubs right now, and I feel great!). If that's your authentic style, wear it like a boss!

The point is that genuine love is not based on achievement or appearance. We will never be more worthy of love than we are at this very moment. So don't care for yourself *any less* today than you would if you were smaller in size. Decorate and celebrate you *today*!

7. The Biological-Psychological-Spiritual Connection

Numerous studies correlate a deeper sense of purpose, greater happiness, and a higher state of overall health in those who have a religious or spiritual practice. Meditation is associated with health benefits as well.

Its practice is tied to stress reduction, which in turn has a positive effect on our bodies systemically. Meditation can be practiced by anyone, with or without an association to a particular religion or spiritual belief.

I'll be candid and share...I get up at 4:00 am every day (give or take 30 minutes) to ensure I get the quiet time I need to read and meditate on Scriptures uninterrupted before my day gets too busy.

There's no way to quantify the growth that has occurred within me since adopting this practice years ago. As I continue growing in a positive way, everyone I teach, serve, and medically treat benefits, because they're getting a better *me*.

Indeed a powerful trickle-down effect occurs when we consistently practice habits that change us for the better, the full extent of which we'll never even know.

Without inner transformation, weight can be lost, regained, then lost and regained again. Most of us know this from personal experience. But when the very essence of who we are transforms, we are no longer that same person.

A diamond cannot return to a state of disordered carbon. A beautiful change has occurred and there's no going back.

We are more than our physical bodies. Set aside time to care for that part of you that *inhabits* your physical body. The benefits go far beyond greater energy. Not only for you but for all who interact with you.

The Teacher said it well: ***The branch cannot bear fruit of itself, except it abide in the vine.***

∽

Summary of NMD Action Step #4
Seven Simple Steps to Live an Energized Life

How can we accomplish our goals and take-charge of our lives unless we are fully energized? Because we are complex beings of various elements, there are multiple ways to fuel our person, several of which are listed above.

Discover the practices that nourish you best and incorporate them into your NMD lifestyle!

NOW MAKE IT YOUR OWN!

THE HOMESTRETCH

What's My Goal Weight?

"How much should I weigh?" I'm often asked.

Gender, body composition, race, genetics, medical history, and family history are all factors that influence our physiology and can't be ignored when we consider what the ideal weight a person should be.

Because of such human variation, there's no *one-size-fits-all* formula or tool (i.e., body mass index, body composition, body fat percentage, etc.) that can provide the answer to this question.

All can be referenced to provide helpful information but shouldn't be relied upon as the sole determining factor in evaluating one's weight-related health status or in setting weight loss goals. Work with your doctor to determine your current health status and to establish your target weight.

In my practice, I emphasize pursuing optimal health rather than a specific number on the scale. I look for reduction, reversal, or a lowered risk of type 2 diabetes, abnormal cholesterol levels, inflammation, hypertension, and heart rate among other factors.

It's also very important that the patient reports an overall improved quality of life and a reduction of medical symptoms (i.e., less pain, improved energy and mood, greater ease in day-to-day function, etc.).

In addition to improved health, let's face it, we all want to maximize our *va-va-voom*! There's nothing's wrong with that. So, our goal weight also includes reaching the point at which we are *personally* satisfied with our bodies.

We must be careful to not aspire to become the size of someone we admire (some actor, model, friend, co-worker, etc.), or to stay stuck in the past by striving to be the size we were *back in the day* (i.e., in high school, college, when we were single, first married, etc.).

Let go of the past and of old expectations. Today is a new day and you are becoming a new person. You are growing in your mindset, habits, and lifestyle in ways you never have before, and your body will transform to reflect this.

Keep an open mind of what that might look like and aspire to the healthiest and best *you* today.

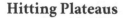

Hitting Plateaus

If your weight loss has stopped before you've reached the weight that best supports optimal health, re-assess your NMD lifestyle. There are likely some Mindset Principles and Action Steps that you have not fully embraced.

Commit to adopting *all* the principles and steps and truly do your best! If you remain plateaued, you may benefit from reading the **MEDICATION** section of this book. If you deem it appropriate, discuss the option of supportive medicinal therapy with your doctor.

Maintenance: A Natural Continuum

Because NMD is a way of life and not a diet, there is no period of restrictive, unsustainable eating in an effort to lose weight, followed by a period called *maintenance* whereby we implement a different way of eating in order to maintain the weight loss.

Eating authentically, being active, and striving to *be better* and to *do better* every day is an ongoing process. There will naturally come a time when weight loss slows down, and the body enters into maintenance.

We do not need to implement any new change in our lifestyle to initiate maintenance or to sustain our weight loss.

~

Make It Your Own!

It's best to establish consistency and stability in practicing the NMD principles and taking the action steps before introducing much change. Once you're firmly rooted in your NMD lifestyle, feel free to branch out a little if you desire. Explore variations of your lifestyle components (e.g., modifying dietary habits, activities, schedules, etc.) until they are optimized to best support your health and weight loss goals.

There is no conflict in incorporating different ideas and strategies into (*but not in place of*) your NMD lifestyle if they enhance it. As you experiment with various tips and suggestions, selectively eliminate those that don't work for you and adopt those that do.

Because we evolve over time, our practices must evolve along with us. So, for ongoing success, we must ultimately develop the confidence to customize our NMD lifestyle according to what is best for us at any given time.

This *your* NMD lifestyle. Make it your own!

~

Before delving into our final section *MEDICATION*, I'm delighted to share one of my favorite testimonials with you.

The next few pages detail a conversation that took place early in my family medicine training. This conversation helped solidify my confidence in the NMD lifestyle and strengthen my resolve to focus my medical practice on obesity treatment.

TESTIMONIAL ~ SIMPLE STEPS, HUGE SUCCESS!

MARIE'S STORY

"*D*r. Collins! Dr. Collins!" I turned around to see Marie, the family practice nurse, bounding toward me full of excitement. I had just returned from lunch and my clinic schedule was full. A full clinic was always challenging for me.

I enjoy taking my time and getting to know my patients. I'll teach and I'll counsel, and I'll listen and learn from them as well. I find that most patients have a lot to share when they know they are valued and the space is provided for a symbiotic relationship.

In family medicine, this is how the patient-doctor relationship develops and how continuity is established.

However, relationship-building takes time and I often got lost in the process. This sometimes resulted in staying after hours; not just myself, but some clinic staff as well. Understandably, this made me a little less popular to work with for some staff.

"We're going to clock out on time today, *riiiiight* Dr. Collins?" "Um, I'll do my best." was all I could promise. And I *would* do my best. But despite my efforts, I rarely finished work on time.

Which is why I was apprehensive about Marie approaching me at the start of clinic. 'No time to talk now!' I thought. 'I need to hit the ground running, so we won't be here late...or *later*...or *later than my usual late*...or something like that.'

So I opened my mouth to politely cut Marie off, but she didn't give me the chance. She began to rave while still a ways off. "Thank you Dr. Collins! Thank you! Thank you! Thank you so much! I just wanted to say thank you!" "For what?" I looked at her, completely puzzled.

"I've lost twenty-two pounds already!" she said. "I'm so excited. It's working. It's really working!"

I flashed back to a conversation we had in that same hallway six or seven weeks earlier when Marie approached me between clinic appointments and asked me how I had lost so much weight. It was the second year of my family medicine training at Kaiser Permanente.

I already knew I wanted to practice bariatric medicine (non-surgical treatment of obesity) upon completing the residency program. I had been my own first NMD patient and had lost over 50 pounds, so I was frequently approached by family, friends, and colleagues, and asked how I lost the weight.

I often found myself counseling people impromptu on the NMD lifestyle, just as I had done with Marie weeks earlier.

Once I realized that Marie was referring to her weight loss success, I was all ears! After all, helping others slay the beast of obesity is what I lived for! So I did away with my commitment to stick to the clinic schedule (there's always tomorrow!). I stopped in my tracks, and joined Marie in her enthusiasm. We were squealing like teenagers just asked to prom!

"Wow, that's great!" I said. "Congratulations!" I think I was more excited than her.

"Can you tell?" She grabbed the waistband of her scrubs and rotated them around her waist – to the right, to the left, and to the right again. "Look how loose my pants are getting!" she exclaimed. Marie was a short, well-rounded gal about five feet no inches tall, 230 pounds or so.

It was obvious that her pants were loose. I looked at her face. It was thinner and she had an absolute *radiance* about her. She was energetic and healthy in her appearance. She was positively glowing.

"You look great!" I almost yelled. "Tell me!" I demanded. "Tell me *exactly* what principles you've been practicing and what steps you've been taking!"

She said, "I've just been doing a few new things every day. I only eat when I'm hungry and I stop eating before I get full. I eat healthier too! A lot more vegetables. My meals are smaller and more balanced. I have so much more energy!"

"I can tell!" I said.

"I eat whatever I want! My family can't believe it! They keep asking me, 'What kind of diet are you on that you can eat *that*?' I tell them, "I'm not on a diet. This is how I eat! This is my new life!" My husband is catching on and even *he* is losing weight!" Marie was completely beaming. Admittedly, so was I.

"I haven't started exercising yet, but I'm more active in all the little ways you suggested. I walk up and down the stairs during the day at work instead of taking the elevator. And I never drive around looking for close parking spaces anymore. I park on the far side of parking lots and walk *all* the way across them to get where I'm going - on purpose! Ha!" she laughed, amused with herself.

"And it's working! I can't believe it's really working! I'm going to be under 200 pounds soon! I haven't been below 200 in years! Thank you so much, Dr. Collins!"

Marie gave me a big hug and that was it for me. Those few minutes in the hallway solidified my confidence in the *No More Dieting* lifestyle!

Upon completing my training, I went directly to work in bariatric medicine. Today I am grateful to have counseled and treated well over 1,000 patients and have helped them to reach their weight loss goals and enjoy improved health!

As much as I love Marie's testimony, I have to admit that every patient's story isn't all rainbows and candy apples. In fact there's a crash and burn story in the next chapter that bears telling if for no other reason than to urge caution.

A WORD OF CAUTION!

ROXANNE'S STORY

As we journey along our transformative path, developing into our best selves yet, we must take caution to protect our growth and guard against that which could dismantle what we have invested our heart and soul into building.

It wasn't until I worked with Roxanne that I realized how critical it is to...

Watch Out for Saboteurs!

Roxanne, a quiet-spoken, warm-hearted woman was a patient of mine in my first year of private practice. She was about 60 pounds overweight and somewhat skeptical that she could lose it without dieting. But because she had never lost it *with dieting*, she figured she would give the NMD lifestyle a chance.

Five weeks later, she was 20 pounds lighter and we were both elated! Until...

During the second month of her NMD lifestyle, Roxanne had an appointment for a physical exam with her primary doctor. During the appointment, her doctor appropriately addressed Roxanne's weight (Rox was obese).

Roxanne enthusiastically explained that she was in the process of losing weight and informed her doctor that she had already lost 20 pounds. Her doctor asked what plan she was doing and Roxanne tried to explain the NMD lifestyle.

Sensing a lack of understanding on her doctor's part, the more Rox spoke, the more uncomfortable she became. As the doctor quietly stared, seemingly unimpressed, Rox began to feel foolish. She began to stammer as she lost confidence in her own words.

The doctor abruptly scoffed when Rox stated she had worked up to exercising 25 minutes a day.

"That's not enough!" the doctor said in a condescending tone. "You need to exercise at least 45 minutes a day to lose weight!"

And that was it. That was all she wrote. Nail in the tire. Roxanne deflated.

Her newly developed confidence didn't have the constitution to hold up against judgement and disapproval from a perceived authority figure. So Roxanne stopped talking and the doctor took over.

Apathetic to Roxanne's weight loss and expanding exercise endurance, the doctor dismissed her success along with her sustainable regimen. She instead robotically regurgitated the same advice that is given to millions of people each year. "Diet and increase your exercise."

She handed Roxanne some version of the same ol' calorie-counting plan she had failed at many times before. But the saddest part is, Rox accepted it without a peep. She had no confidence that the diet would work for her, but she felt too intimidated to say so.

I'm not sure who I was more frustrated with, Rox or her doctor. Because despite outstanding progress and clear evidence of what was working for her in contrast to what previously hadn't, Roxanne allowed negative, outside influence to infiltrate her new mindset and to sabotage her success.

In the following weeks, Roxanne failed the diet. She wasn't able to exercise to the extent the doctor wanted, so she stopped exercising altogether.

Predictably, she began steadily regaining her weight. In contrast to the happy, hopeful, energetic person she had started to become, whenever I spoke with her, she sounded depressed. I tried to convince her to break out of her rut by resuming the NMD lifestyle and to be honest with her doctor about doing so, and why. But she declined. She was firmly rooted in regression.

How I wished Roxanne would have stayed the course long enough to experience real change! But instead, she chose to pursue outside approval and validation above her own obvious good.So I made myself available to her should she ever change her mind, and I moved on.

Dear reader, please watch out for saboteurs! Even those who mean well. Protect your NMD lifestyle from the doubters and naysayers. Don't allow the opinions of others to lure you away from what's working, back to what you have tried and failed numerous times. **You know what they say about insanity...** But I'm confident that *you* will stay the course! So let's move on.

It's time to get down to the nitty gritty and break down the topic of MEDICATION.

Ready? Good!

Come with me...

MEDICATION

IS PRESCRIPTION MEDICATION THE MISSING PIECE OF THE PUZZLE FOR YOU?

MEDICATION

INTRODUCTION

Most people can reach their weight loss goal just by adopting the NMD lifestyle alone. However, some people benefit more when weight loss medication is added to their efforts. The reason for this varies.

Some have overwhelming food cravings or struggle significantly with impulse control. Many have been steeped in compulsive eating and/or binge eating so long that additional support is needed during the process of releasing old beliefs and habits while adopting healthier ones. Still, others may battle metabolic disease, psychiatric disease, or any combination of issues.

Regardless of the reason, overweight and obese people who have not been able to successfully lose weight on their own should be aware that there is help available by means of weight loss medication.

When such people meet the criteria to be treated with medication, and the potential benefit of treating outweighs the risk, the option of treatment should be presented by their doctor and discussed with the patient. Unfortunately, this is rarely the case.

∽

The controversy surrounding obesity treatment (*or the lack thereof*) is worthy of extended discussion.

Please lend me an ear as we forge this largely untrodden terrain here in *MEDICATION*.

∽

There are 3 parts that make-up MEDICATION

- Let's Talk About It

- Med Lists, Disclaimers, and Discussions

- All FDA-Approved Medications Discussed in Detail

Let's begin...

LET'S TALK ABOUT IT

MEDICATION

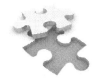

TO MEDICATE, OR NOT MEDICATE.
THAT IS THE QUESTION...

*O*besity is the fastest-growing cause of disease and death in the United States. A staggering 1 out of every 8 deaths caused by illness is directly related to being overweight/obese.

The rate of obesity has increased to the point that the number of obese Americans is now greater than the number of overweight Americans. Even worse, obesity (or *globesity,* shall we say?) is now a global epidemic.

In light of the devastation that's associated with obesity, it's hard to justify treating numerous obesity-related diseases while being passive about treating the core issue itself, which arguably has been the standard medical practice for years.

This is not to say doctors are all to blame. I can't count the number of obese patients I've had who take medication for several conditions such as hypertension, type 2 diabetes, abnormal cholesterol levels, depression, anxiety, or chronic pain., Additionally, they haven't been able to lose weight on their own. Yet, when I initiate a discussion about treating their obesity with lifestyle counseling *and medication*, the patient adamantly declines. "No! I don't want to rely on a crutch!" they'll say, referring to the weight loss medication.

Curiously, a few of my heaviest patients rely on walkers to help support their body weight when they walk. Some have surrendered altogether to electric wheelchairs. But the same people may decline medication that could help them lose the weight because to take the medication would be *"relying on a crutch."*

Does anyone else see the irony?

Obesity is a disease-loaded machine gun. Is it really more sensible to take its continuous hits and chronically patch-up the wounds with a plethora of medicine for chronic disease (usually taken for life), rather than to *disable the weapon*?

It's critical to make the distinction between medication treatment for obesity-related *chronic disease* versus medication treatment for *obesity itself*. The endpoint is quite different.

Medicine for chronic disease (i.e., type 2 diabetes, hypertension, dyslipidemia, etc.) is prescribed for the purpose of disease *management,* not cure. Patients are usually prescribed these medications and take them for the remainder of their life to help stabilize chronic disease.

Medicine for weight loss is prescribed for the purpose of *disease reversal*. Patients who lose their excess weight are reversing obesity. Additionally, reversing obesity usually results in reversing (or at least *reducing*) the obesity-related diseases as well.

This usually necessitates a reduction or discontinuation of the medications the patient is taking to manage these diseases **(read the chapter on how Orlando reversed metabolic syndrome for a prime example of this)**.

So why do we accept lifetime treatment for chronic disease, but shun obesity treatment which can lead to the reversal of not just obesity, but obesity-related diseases as well?

∼

The Obesity Stigma

Many in society, including healthcare workers and patients, have long considered obesity solely the consequence of those who lack self-control and execute poor judgment in their life-style choices. Indeed a stigma of laziness, flawed character, and even one of lacking morality is associated with being obese.

Asking for help to lose weight is perceived as not taking responsibility for one's own behavior, using medication is seen as a *weakness*, and the medication itself is considered a *crutch*. Conversely, faithfully seeking medical care to manage obesity-related conditions (and other conditions) is considered *responsible*.

Why the double standard?

The obesity stigma *lays blame* on the overweight/obese person for their condition. *They got themselves into this mess, let them get themselves out of it!* is often the unspoken sentiment.

However, obesity can't be reduced to just a *voluntary condition* that developed by way of poor choices. Lifestyle choices are a major contributor, but they're not the *only* contributor.

The cause of obesity is multifactorial, or as stated by The Obesity Society (TOS) *"Obesity is a complex condition with numerous causes, many of which are largely beyond an individual's control."*

Laying aside the issue of *cause*, let's dispel the myth that those who receive medication treatment will have less responsibility in taking the necessary steps to lose weight.

In fact, if a patient doesn't adopt healthy lifestyle habits, such as those outlined in NMD, any weight that was lost while taking the medication will most likely be regained once the medication is discontinued.

For this reason, it is imperative that *lifestyle change* be the emphasis of any weight loss treatment plan and not the medication. The medication serves only to *supplement* the patient's own weight loss efforts; it cannot replace them.

It is not a magic bullet nor a quick-fix. But for some, the medication proves to be an immensely supportive element that fills in the gap between the patient's best efforts and the point of successfully reaching their goal weight.

MEDICATION

An example of this would be...

MY PERSONAL EXPERIENCE WITH WEIGHT LOSS MEDICATION

I have always been very candid about my own personal experience with NMD and the use of prescription weight loss medication. The reason I am so open about it is so that those who struggle with losing weight will be encouraged and know that they too can reverse obesity and overcome compulsive eating.

In the introduction of this book, I told you *My Story and the Birth of No More Dieting*. To be specific, I relayed how the *MIND* and *MOTION* components of NMD came to be. **The mindset principles in MIND and the action steps in MOTION are the essential and indispensable core components of NMD.**

The remainder of this chapter depicts the conclusion of my weight loss journey and how the *MEDICATION* component of NMD came to be.

Note: The *MEDICATION* component of NMD is *optional* and won't be needed for most people who have adopted the NMD lifestyle.

~

The Conclusion of My Weight Loss Journey

After having my second baby, I lost about 40 pounds just by adopting the NMD lifestyle (see *My Story and the Birth of NMD*).

I then hit a plateau and remained stuck for a while without losing weight. I was already a doctor at this time, so it was logical for me to turn to science and research to see what was successfully being done to treat the obese and overweight population.

After learning my options, I decided I would pursue medicinal treatment (prescription medication) to supplement my weight loss efforts. I went prepared with data in hand to see my primary care doctor, who happened to be newly assigned to me.

I brought an obesity treatment guide published by the National Institutes of Health (NIH) to my appointment, because in my experience most doctors are not very knowledgeable about treatment with weight loss medication and they tend to be very resistant to prescribing it.

During my exam, my doctor and I chatted, getting to know each other. I soon began sharing my history of obesity, a lifetime of diet failures, and how I had recently lost a lot of weight by adopting a healthier mindset and by taking action steps.

She was thrilled to hear it! I went on to explain how despite my recent efforts, I had not been able to make any further weight loss progress. I then asked if she would support my health and wellness goals by prescribing an appetite suppressant to supplement my continued weight loss efforts.

I might here mention that my doctor was thin. She freely admitted she had never had a "weight problem" and that she couldn't relate to the struggle.

I appreciated that she was so open and willing to have a dialogue about it. She also acknowledged that she didn't know anything about the *pharmacological* treatment of obesity (beyond the dreadful *Fen-Phen* era, which is discussed in the chapter on Phentermine).

As anticipated, she was resistant to treating me, not because she wasn't supportive, but because she was largely ignorant regarding effective treatment for overweight/obese patients. But that was okay because I had come prepared to respectfully argue my case.

I showed her the data and was cautiously optimistic when she sat down and quietly read the parts of the report I had carefully highlighted. Every minute or so she'd turn the page and thoughtfully scan it from top to bottom.

It seemed like an eternity as I waited for her verdict. Thankfully, by the end of my appointment, my doctor had agreed to prescribe a 30-day supply of an appetite suppressant (medically called *anorectant, anorectic* or *anorexiant* medication) to help support my weight loss efforts. But I would need to follow-up with her before she would grant any refills. I was grateful that she was willing to venture outside of her comfort zone, and I assured her I would follow-up as she requested.

A month later, with my continued NMD lifestyle and the added pharmacological support, I had lost another 6 pounds and a dress size, which had been my typical monthly weight loss prior to hitting the plateau. I reported this to my doctor who was very pleased.

Surprisingly, she thanked me! She said she was now more knowledgeable and better equipped to treat overweight and obese patients. Needless to say, she readily refilled my prescription.

Once I reached my goal weight, I stopped taking the medication. I had permanently adopted the NMD lifestyle so I easily maintained my 50+ pound weight loss and still continue to do so.

NO GUILT! NO SHAME!

*C*ommitting to lifestyle change is the *fundamental prescription* for permanent weight loss and improved health.

This is accomplished in a painless, doable way with the NMD lifestyle, which is adaptable to begin immediately, at any starting point, and for all people. However, some people continue struggling to lose weight despite their best efforts.

If this is true for you, don't hesitate to discuss your challenges with your doctor and to carefully consider the options that are available to you. Weigh the potential risks and benefits of accepting medicinal help versus the risks and benefits of declining it. Then make the decision that best suits you.

Do not entertain thoughts of failure, guilt, or shame if you decide to accept medicinal help.

Regardless of the choice you make, continue striving daily to improve your NMD lifestyle, for this is the essential path to permanent weight loss and weight maintenance.

That being said, it's time we get down to the meat and potatoes (so to speak) of weight-loss medication.

Here we go...

MED LISTS, DISCLAIMERS, AND DISCUSSIONS

In this section we'll discuss the following topics:

- Disclaimer
- Criteria for Treatment with Prescription Weight Loss Medicine
- Current FDA-Approved Prescription Weight Loss Medications
- **New in 2019 - FDA-Approved Oral Weight Management Device**
- Phentermine; Guilty by Association
- Off-Label Prescribing, Combo Meds, and Meds for Longterm Use
- Anorectant medications and DEA schedules

DISCLAIMER

*B*efore discussing today's FDA-approved weight loss medications in the following chapters, we have some less-stimulating, albeit necessary business to tend to...

~

DISCLAIMER

This book includes brief, very general discussions about various medications and an oral device used for weight loss and weight management respectively. The information in this book is limited and does not include the majority of information about the possible uses, directions, warnings, precautions, contraindications, drug-interactions, adverse events, side-effects, risks, specific criteria for treatment, etc.

For more information about FDA-approved medications, visit the Food and Drug Administration website at: www.fda.gov.

The information presented in this book is to provide awareness only. It is not medical advice and should not be mistaken as medical advice, nor should this information be used to decide whether or not to take any of these or other medications or weight management aids.

By reading the contents of this book, you acknowledge and agree that the information therein may contain inaccuracies and/or other errors. Your reliance upon information and content in this book is solely at your own risk.

See your doctor, or licensed healthcare provider before adopting any dietary, exercise, medicinal, or supplemental changes or practices.

This information does not endorse any medicine as safe, effective, or approved for treating any person or health condition. Your health care provider will help you decide if medication therapy is right for you.

The content of this book does not replace information you receive from your health care provider. You must talk with your healthcare provider for complete information about the risks and benefits of using these or any medications or weight management aids.

Your medical provider is responsible for independently reaching any medical judgment and for any resulting diagnosis and treatments, in spite of any use of this book's content by your medical professional. Readers are solely responsible for their use of this content.

The author does not assume any liability or responsibility for any damage, injury, or death to you, other persons, or property arising from any use of any information, idea, or instruction contained within the contents of this book.

Before taking any medication or aids, including over-the-counter supplements, talk to your doctor about potential side effects, contraindications, allergic reactions, drug interactions, the possible need for laboratory screening, and whether or not the medication is right for you.

Do not take any medicine or aids (prescription or over the counter) if you are pregnant or nursing unless directed by your physician to do so. The weight-loss medications and weight management device discussed in there book may harm unborn babies. Women who are pregnant should not take these drugs or use the weight management device. Women who do take weight-loss medication or use the weight management devices should avoid getting pregnant.

Whew! Glad that's over. That was exhausting!

Now we can get started...

CRITERIA FOR TREATMENT WITH PRESCRIPTION WEIGHT LOSS MEDICINE

*G*enerally, prescription weight loss medication is approved for use based body mass index (BMI) which is an index that relates weight to height. Those with a BMI of 30 or greater (obesity), *or* those with a BMI of 27 or greater (overweight) if they also have at least one weight-related medical condition such as type 2 diabetes, hypertension, or dyslipidemia (abnormal cholesterol levels) will usually qualify for treatment with prescription weight loss medicine.

The BMI to use Plenity, an FDA-approved weight management device is 27 (**for details see *New in 2019 - FDA-Approved Oral Weight management Device**)

That being said, there are many people who need treatment, but may not meet the stated criteria. To these I suggest meeting with your healthcare provider to discuss your particular challenges.

In light of the staggering degree of morbidity and mortality surrounding obesity and its associated diseases, I emphasize to medical providers how critical it is to fully consider the risk versus the benefit of prescribing weight loss medicine versus not prescribing.

Using their discretion, providers must consider each patient uniquely and ultimately provide the treatment that's in the best interest of the patient. Sometimes, this means crafting a treatment plan that doesn't fall within traditional guidelines.

CURRENT FDA-APPROVED PRESCRIPTION WEIGHT LOSS MEDICATIONS AND AN ORAL DEVICE

*T*oday's FDA-Approved Weight Loss Medications and an Oral Weight Management Device

Eleven medications and one oral device are currently FDA-approved for weight loss and weight management respectively. The medications are listed here in alphabetical order by their generic name, with a common brand-name in parenthesis. The oral weight management device follows.

Please note that some medications have more than one brand-name, or are available in different forms, or by different means of delivery (i.e. capsules, tables, slow-release, extended release, etc.). Such details are not included here.

Each medication and the oral device will be discussed in detail in subsequent chapters and in the Medication section: *All FDA-Approved Medications and An Oral Device Discussed in Detail*

∼

The 11 FDA-Approved Weight Loss Medications

1. Amphetamine sulfate (Evekeo)
2. Benzphetamine (Didrex)
3. Contrave (Naltrexone SR/ Bupropion SR)
4. Diethylpropion (Tenuate, Dospan)
5. Liraglutide (Saxenda)
6. Lorcaserin (Belviq)
7. Methamphetamine (Desoxyn)
8. Orlistat (Xenical, Alli)
9. Phendimetrazine (Bontril)
10. Phentermine (Adipex-P)
11. Qsymia (Phentermine/Topiramate ER)

∼

*New in 2019: There is 1 FDA-Approved Oral Weight Management Device

1. Plenity

Plenity is discussed in detail in the chapter entitled *New in 2019 - FDA-Approved Oral Weight management Device.*

In the following chapters we'll discuss each medication and the device individually as well as categorize and discuss them within groups to learn about them from different perspectives.

But before we proceed, we must take a moment to address a few historical rumors that have unduly tainted the reputation of all weight loss medications indiscriminately, potentially impeding millions of people from getting the care they need.

Although a touchy subject for some, this discussion is unavoidable. We *have* to go there.

So gird up and let's go...

PHENTERMINE

GUILTY BY ASSOCIATION

It all started in the 90's...

In 1992, two different appetite suppressants, Fenfluramine and Phentermine were combined, producing an amplified anorectant effect (loss of appetite).

This combination called Fen-Phen was heavily marketed, and its popularity spread like wildfire.

However, there were reports about an association between Fenfluramine and the rare, but potentially fatal pulmonary hypertension.

As an alternative medication, the chemically similar drug Dexfenfluramine was produced by the same company that produced Fenfluramine. Nevertheless, cases of pulmonary hypertension continued to occur.

In 1996, cases of cardiac valve disease in patients who had taken Fen-Phen began to be publicized.

More and more cases of heart valve disease and pulmonary hypertension emerged, until the FDA withdrew Fenfluramine, Dexfenfluramine, and the Fen-Phen combination medication from the market in 1997.

That same year, the Centers for Disease Control and Prevention (CDC) publicized a detailed article entitled "Cardiac Valvulopathy Associated with Exposure to Fenfluramine or Dexfenfluramine..." in which it stated that heart valve disease developed in patients who had taken either Fenfluramine alone, Dexfenfluramine alone; a combination of Fenfluramine and Phentermine; or a combination of all three drugs. "None of the cases used phentermine alone."

It is important to point out that Phentermine, the most frequently prescribed weight loss medicine world-wide, has been in use for over 55 years (FDA-approved in 1959). In fact, it had been in use for over 30 years before being combined with fenfluramine and dexfenfluramine and it was never labeled as a cause of heart and lung disease.

Appropriately, Phentermine was not recalled by the FDA and continues to be prescribed to millions of patients each year.

But unfortunately, it was widely reported that 'weight loss drugs cause heart disease' without any distinction between the guilty drugs versus the innocent.

Since the Fen-Phen era, despite the rising rate of obesity, doctors have been afraid to treat obesity with weight loss medicine and patients have been afraid to be treated.

Another myth that has hindered overweight and obese people from receiving safe medicinal treatment, is the belief that *all weight loss pills are addictive.* This is simply not true.

The International Journal of Obesity and Related Metabolic Disorders published an article in 2014 entitled *Addiction Potential of Phentermine Prescribed During Long-Term Treatment of Obesity* in which it concluded "**Phentermine abuse or psychological dependence (addiction) does not occur in patients treated with phentermine for obesity.**" This included patients who were taking higher Phentermine doses, and who had taken it for extended periods of time.

Generally, addictive behavior can be characterized by continually seeking out the substance (e.g. drugs, etc.) or behavior (e.g. gambling, etc.) to which a person is addicted. The behavior will escalate despite significant negative consequences, such as loss of employment, destruction of relationships, loss of financial security, etc. **This is not known to occur with the most commonly prescribed weight loss medications.**

That being said, there are some less frequently prescribed weight loss medications that *do* have a higher potential for abuse. We will touch upon them later when we discuss *scheduled medication.*

There are numerous studies and reports that affirm the relative safety of Phentermine (when taken as directed). In fact Qsymia, a combination weight loss medication that includes Phentermine, was FDA-approved in 2012 for long-term (potentially life-long) use.

Undoubtedly, more approved Phentermine-combos will follow, as bariatricians have been prescribing Phentermine and Phentermine-combos off label for decades. Their safety has been documented and the logical need for them is finally being recognized.

Let's talk more about off-label prescribing, combination medications, and medication for longterm use.

Come with me to the next chapter...

OFF-LABEL PRESCRIBING, COMBO MEDS & MEDS FOR LONGTERM USE

*O*ff-Label Use of Medicine for Weight Loss

The term *off-label* is applied when medicine or therapy is prescribed for a purpose, or for a period of time that it has not been approved by the FDA. This practice is legal and very common among medical providers.

A recognizable example of this is when aspirin (or "baby aspirin") is prescribed to help prevent first-time heart attacks and stroke, usually in the older population. But actually, aspirin is not FDA-approved for primary prevention of heart attacks and stroke.

Next time you're in a drug store, grab a bottle of aspirin off the shelf and take a careful look at the label. You may see a 'heart' that the manufacturer put on the box to imply that the medication is for cardiac health, but the label will read 'pain reliever' because this is what aspirin is *officially* approved to treat by the FDA.

Other examples of off-label treatment are: anti-seizure medicine prescribed for depression, antidepressant medication prescribed for chronic pain, and allergy medicine prescribed for cold symptoms.

Off-label prescribing as a part of obesity treatment includes prescribing medication that is FDA-approved to treat other conditions (e.g. depression, seizure, type 2 diabetes, or prediabetes, etc.). Such medications are often used because of their known side effect of weight loss.

The 4 medications listed below are not FDA-approved as weight loss medications when prescribed as a singular medicine (i.e. not as part of a combo-medicine). Nevertheless, they have been prescribed *off-label* as single agents for weight loss for many years.

Examples of medication that are FDA-approved for other conditions but commonly prescribed off-label for weight loss:

- Bupropion (Wellbutrin) an antidepressant
- Metformin (Glucophage) an antihyperglycemic
- Naltrexone, low dose (LDN) an opiate antagonist
- Topiramate (Topamax) an antiepileptic

Interestingly, after many years of off-label use, several of these medications were incorporated into combination weight loss pills. As such, they are now FDA-approved for weight loss, but only when taken as part of the combination pills (see below).

FDA-Approved Weight Loss Combination Medications

- Qsymia (Phentermine/Topiramate ER)
- Contrave (Naltrexone SR/ Bupropion SR)

As noted above, three of the four medications (Topiramate, Naltrexone, and Bupropion) that make up the two combination medications Qsymia and Contrave, have been commonly used off-label (as singular-medication) for many years because of their well-known side effect of weight loss.

Fun Fact: Phentermine is also usually used off-label because it is almost always prescribed beyond the FDA-approved treatment period of "a few weeks."

Phentermine has been prescribed in combination with other medications as off-label weight loss therapy for years. One combination is Phentermine with a relatively low dose of the antidepressant medication Prozac.

This combination is referred to as Phen-Pro. Prozac is in a class of medication called selective serotonin reuptake inhibitors (SSRIs). When taken in combination with Phentermine, Prozac is thought to enhance the anorectic effect, and reduce/delay the tolerance of Phentermine so that it continues to be effective long-term.

Historically, a warning of the rare, but potentially fatal serotonin syndrome exists when combining Phentermine with SSRIs. But this thought has been challenged in studies and by frequent prescribers of Phen-Pro.

For instance, Dr. Michael Anchors, a seasoned bariatrician and pioneer of the Phen-Pro regimen, authored a book about it called *Safer Than Phen-Fen!* Dr. Anchors has treated thousands of patients with the Phen-Pro combination, including at least 15 who lost over 100 pounds. Dr. Anchords is a vocal advocate of the safety and effectiveness of its use, not only for weight loss, but for ongoing maintenance if needed.

FDA-Approved Weight Loss Medications and One Weight Management Device for Chronic (Potentially Lifetime) Use

The medications listed below have been FDA-approved for lifetime use if the patient meets the criteria to take them and is losing weight while on them.

- Contrave (Naltrexone SR/ Bupropion SR)
- Liraglutide (Saxenda)
- Lorcaserin (Belviq)
- Orlistat (Xenical; Alli)
- Qsymia (Phentermine/Topiramate ER)

There is One Orally-Administered Weight Management Device that is FDA-Approved for Longterm Use

- Plenity

For details about Plenity, see the chapter entitled *New in 2019 - FDA-Approved Oral Weight management Device

Let's head over to the next chapter to breakdown DEA Schedules and discuss how weight loss medicine fits into this system.

See you there!

DEA SCHEDULED ANORECTANT MEDICATION

*A*norectants, also known as anorexiant, anorexigenic, and anorectic medication, are drugs that result in weight loss primarily by suppressing appetite.

These medications work by affecting neurotransmitters (chemical messengers) in the central nervous system. In essence, they effect the brain's chemistry resulting in the suppression of hunger.

Some anorectics are associated with having an increased metabolic effect and breaking down fat. Additionally, many people report a significant reduction in cravings while taking anorectants.

Anorectants are stimulant medications which can produce a sense of euphoria, potentially making them more addictive then medication that does not produce such an effect.

Medications that have addictive properties are labeled as controlled medications or *substances.*

Controlled medications are assigned to one of five drug schedules (categories) with Schedule 1 drugs having the highest abuse potential (Schedule 1 drugs are not prescribed at all for medical use in the US), through Schedule 5 drugs, which have the lowest abuse potential.

See the summary below.

For more details regarding DEA controlled substance schedules visit: www.deadiversion.usdoj.gov/schedules/#define

There are 8 FDA-approved anorectant medications that are assigned to schedules

As of the writing of this book, there are 8 FDA-approved anorectant medications that are assigned to schedules ranging from Schedule 2 (high abuse potential) through Schedule 4 (relatively low abuse potential). These medications are listed below. Each will be discussed in detail in the final section of this book *All FDA-Approved Medications Discussed in Detail.*

1. Schedule 1 Substances: High potential for abuse

There are currently no Schedule 1 drugs that are used in medical practice in the US.

2. Schedule 2 Anorectics: High potential for abuse; may lead to severe psychological or physical dependence.

• Amphetamine sulfate (Evekeo)

• Methamphetamine (Desoxyn)

3. Schedule 3 Anorectics: Potential for abuse is less than drugs in Schedules 1 and 2; abuse may lead to low to moderate physical dependence or high psychological dependence.

• Benzphetamine (Didrex)

• Phendimetrazine (Bontril)

4. Schedule 4 Anorectics: Low potential for abuse (relative to Schedule 3 substances).

• Lorcaserin (Belviq)

• Phentermine (Adipex-P)

• Phentermine/Topiramate-ER (Qsymia)

• Diethylpropion (Tenuate, Dospan)

5. Schedule 5 Substances: Low potential for abuse (relative to Schedule 4 substances).

There are no Schedule 5 weight loss medications

Regarding scheduled medications, I tend to prescribe the lowest scheduled weight loss medications which fall into Schedule 4. This is not just because of their relatively low abuse potential, but because my patients are counseled with NMD, which places the emphasis on immediate and consistent life-style improvement which naturally leads to weight loss.

It's time to enter into our final MEDICATION section where you will learn in detail all you want (and more than you need) about every weight loss medication listed in this book.

So pour yourself a big cup o' joe and I'll see you there...

ALL FDA-APPROVED MEDICATION AND AN ORAL DEVICE DISCUSSED IN DETAIL

In this section we'll discuss all medications and one oral device in detail. We will cover:

- Current FDA-approved weight loss medications
- *New in 2019: FDA-Approved Oral Weight Management Device
- The individual components of FDA-approved combination drugs as well as the combination drugs as a whole.
- FDA-approved weight loss medications and aids that are approved for longterm use.
- Medications that are not FDA-approved for weight loss but are commonly prescribed *off-label* for weight loss.

Let's first define the term 'black box warning' because you will see it in association with some drugs.

Boxed (also known as black box) warnings on drug labels are required by the FDA for drugs that have a significant risk of resulting in very serious, or even life-threatening adverse events.

I think we're ready so let's get started...

FDA-APPROVED WEIGHT LOSS MEDS, COMBO MEDS, AND MEDS FOR LONGTERM USE

*T*here are 11 FDA-approved weight loss medications. They are listed in alphabetical order below and discussed in detail.

#1 Amphetamine sulfate (Evekeo)

Evekeo is an amphetamine anorectic, which is **absolutely not commonly used for weight loss**.

Evekeo is a Schedule 2 controlled substance, meaning it's among the FDA-approved drugs with the highest addition and abuse potential.

It was FDA-approved in 2012, although amphetamine has been FDA-approved for decades to treat other medical conditions (e.g. ADHD, narcolepsy, etc.).

Evekeo is approved for obesity treatment for a very limited time (a few weeks) and in refractory cases only.

I have never had the need to prescribe this drug, nor do I know any bariatricians who have used it.

It's reasonable to assume that the potential harm in using this drug may outweigh the medical benefit in all but extreme circumstances.

Evekeo has a **BLACK BOX WARNING**, a portion of which states:

Amphetamines have a high potential for abuse; taking amphetamines for prolonged periods may lead to drug dependence; misuse of amphetamine may cause sudden death and serious cardiovascular adverse events.

FOR THE COMPLETE BLACK BOX WARNING VISIT: www.Evekeo.com

~

#2 Benzphetamine (Didrex)

Benzphetamine is a sympathomimetic amine anorectic. It is a Schedule 3 controlled substance, meaning as defined by the DEA it has "a potential for abuse less than substances in Schedules 1 or 2; abuse may lead to moderate or low physical dependence or high psychological dependence."

Generally, I take this to mean that Schedule 3 drugs have a moderate potential for abuse and dependency, relative to the other scheduled drugs.

Benzphetamine was FDA-approved in 1960.

Currently, I would not say that this medication is frequently prescribed, compared to other FDA-approved weight loss medications.

~

#3 Contrave (Naltrexone SR/ Bupropion SR)

Contrave is a combination of the two drugs Naltrexone and Bupropion. It was FDA-approved in 2014. It is not a Scheduled medication (not a controlled substance).

Naltrexone is used to treat opioid and alcohol dependence. Bupropion is an antidepressant, and is also prescribed for smoking cessation. Both of these medications have been prescribed off-label for weight loss for many years.

Together, they are thought to have a synergistic effect. More details about each medication is provided separately in the chapter *FDA-Approved Meds Used Off-Label for Weight Loss*.

Contrave is one of the four medications that have been FDA-approved in recent years for chronic, even lifelong use if needed. The other three were approved prior to Contrave; they are Orlistat, Belviq, and Qsymia.

Contrave might be a good weight loss medication option for patients who would also benefit from treatment for either depression, smoking cessation, opioid abuse, and/or alcohol abuse. Discuss this with your doctor if you think this is true for you.

Contrave has a **BLACK BOX WARNING, a portion of which states:**

Antidepressants have an increased risk of suicidal thoughts and behaviors changes associated with their use.

Because Contrave contains the antidepressant Bupropion, a boxed warning is warranted. Additionally, serious neuropsychiatric events have occurred in patients taking Bupropion for smoking cessation.

Do not drink alcohol or take opioids while taking Contrave. If you have been taking opioid medicine for an extended period of time, tell your doctor.

You may need to be off opioid medication for at least 7-10 days before starting Contrave.

FOR THE COMPLETE BLACK BOX WARNING VISIT:

www.Contrave.com

~

#4 Diethylpropion (Tenuate, Tenuate Dospan-controlled release)

Tenuate (let's use the brand name) is a sympathomimetic amine anorectic. It is a Schedule 4 controlled substance, meaning it has low potential for abuse (relative to Schedule 3 drugs).

Tenuate has been FDA-approved since 1959. Currently, I would not say that it is commonly prescribed, compared to other FDA-approved weight loss medications. However, I have prescribed it quite a bit.

Generally, my patients report that Tenuate has a more subtle effect than Phentermine (which I prescribe most often).

So I find it to be an excellent option for patients who are sensitive to stimulants, (such as those with low tolerance to caffeine).

I also consider it beneficial that Tenuate is taken three times a day. This allows the patient some control over the frequency and intensity of side effects.

For example, the prescription can be written such that patients can choose to skip a dose if it's not needed. So if they don't need appetite control in the morning, they can just take the afternoon and evening doses. Or, if they opt to skip the evening dose to avoid insomnia (a common side effect for most anorectics), they can do so.

Taking two-thirds of the daily dose in this manner would reduce side effects, but on the flip side it would also reduce the desired effect of overall appetite suppression. Finding the optimal balance between desired medication effect and unwanted side effects is always a treatment goal. Fortunately, with all the weight loss medications and dosing options, this is not difficult to do.

To be clear, the above is referring to Tenuate, which is an immediate-release tablet that's taken three times a day prior to meals.

Diethylpropion is also available as Tenuate Dospan, which is a higher-dose, controlled-release tablet that is taken once daily.

~

#5 Liraglutide (Saxenda)

Liraglutide is in a class of medications called incretin mimetics. It is not a Scheduled medication (not a controlled substance).

Liraglutide was FDA-approved in 2010 *as Victoza* to treat type 2 diabetes. Later, in 2014 (with different dosing) it was FDA-approved as Saxenda for long-term weight loss treatment and weight management.

Liraglutide works by mimicking the action of a naturally occurring hormone (an incretin) in the body called GLP-1 (glucagon-like peptide-1).

GLP-1 regulates blood sugar by stimulating insulin secretion and suppressing glucagon when blood sugar levels rise. It also helps control hunger by slowing the stomach-emptying process.

Liraglutide is the first medication in its class to gain FDA-approval for the purpose of weight loss. It's approved for chronic weight management, life-long if needed.

Conceptually, this drug seems ideal for obese/overweight patients with type 2 diabetes, which are many. However, there are a few issues surrounding Liraglutide that make it less appealing to prescribers and patients alike.

Most concerning is its serious black box warning (see below). Less concerning, but still a problem for some, is that the drug is self-injected by the patient once a day via a pre-filled injection pen.

A huge hindrance for many patients is the medication cost of over $1000 per month. That's with insurance!

There are many discount cards and payment assistance programs easily found on the internet.

Saxenda has a **BLACK BOX WARNING, a portion of which states:**

Thyroid C-cell tumors developed in rodents studies with Saxenda. It is not known whether Saxenda causes thyroid C-cell tumors, including medullary thyroid carcinoma (MTC) in humans.

Saxenda should not be used in patients with a personal or family history of MTC or in patients with multiple endocrine neoplasia (MEN) syndrome type 2.

FOR THE COMPLETE BLACK BOX WARNING VISIT:

www.Saxenda.com

~

#6 Lorcaserin (Belviq)

Lorcaserin is a scrotonin receptor agonist. It works by changing the chemistry in the brain, ultimately promoting satiety (a sense of fullness in the gut).

Lorcaserin is a Schedule 4 controlled substance, meaning it has low potential for abuse (relative to Schedule 3 drugs). It was FDA-approved in 2012 for *long-term* weight management; life-long if needed.

Fun Fact: Lorcaserin was the first weight loss medication to be FDA-approved after a dry spell of 13 years during which time no new weight loss drugs were approved.

Prior to Lorcaserin, Orlistat (Alli is the OTC, lower-dose version of Orlistat; see below) had been the last weight loss drug approved in 1999.

As possible evidence of the evolving mindset regarding chronic obesity and the need to treat it, Qsymia was approved the month after Lorcaserin. Contrave and Saxenda were approved a couple years later.

All of these medications are approved for long-term weight loss.

~

#7 **Methamphetamine (Desoxyn)**

Desoxyn is a methamphetamine anorectic which is *absolutely not commonly used for weight loss*.

Desoxyn is a Schedule 2 controlled substance, meaning it's among the FDA-approved drugs with the highest addition and abuse potential.

It was FDA-approved in 1943 for obesity treatment for a very limited time (a few weeks) and in refractory cases only.

I have never had the need to prescribe this drug, nor do I know any bariatricians who have used it.

It's reasonable to assume that the potential harm in using this drug may outweigh the medical benefit in all but extreme circumstances.

Desoxyn has a **BLACK BOX WARNING**, a portion of which states:

Methamphetamine has a high potential for abuse. It should thus be tried only in weight reduction programs for patients in whom alternative therapy has been ineffective.

Administration of methamphetamine for prolonged periods of time in obesity may lead to drug dependence and must be avoided. Misuse of methamphetamine may cause sudden death and serious cardiovascular adverse events.

FOR THE COMPLETE BLACK BOX WARNING VISIT:

www.FDA.gov

~

#8 Orlistat (Xenical, Alli)

Xenical (Orlistat 120 mg) was FDA-approved in 1999 and is available by prescription only. Alli (Orlistat 60 mg) was FDA-approved in 2007 and can be purchased over-the-counter (OTC) by adults. Orlistat is not a Scheduled medication (not a controlled substance).

Orlistat works in the intestines as a lipase inhibitor (*fat blocker*), ultimately preventing about 25% of the fat in your meals from being absorbed. The calorie-dense nutrient (aka fat) passes through your intestines and comes out in your stool.

Fun Fact: Alli is the only OTC weight loss drug ever approved by the FDA. Also, it was the last weight loss medication approved before a dry spell of 13 years with no new medication approvals. Then Belviq and Qsymia came on the scene in 2012. During the 13 years, Orlistat was also the only medication approved for long-term use. Now there are several.

Not So Fun Fact: *No more than 30% of the calories in your meals should come from fat* Alli manufacturers warn, and rightfully so. The more fat you eat, the more remains in your gut.

This may lead to an *anal sphincter security breach*, if you will. With any internal pressure - a cough, a sneeze, a laugh - a dignity violation can occur by means of unexpected, oily stool leakage. I'll say no more.

Alli works well. Maybe too well for some, but it does work nonetheless. Successful Allitarians are those who learn (quickly!) to respect the efficacy of the drug and to follow the recommendations. In this way the *Alli-oops* can be avoided.

For more information visit: www.myalli.com

~

#9 Phendimetrazine (Bontril)

Phendimetrazine is a sympathomimetic amine anorectic. It is a Schedule 3 controlled substance, meaning as defined by the DEA it has "a potential for abuse less than substances in Schedules 1 or 2; abuse may lead to moderate or low physical dependence or high psychological dependence."

Generally, I take this to mean that Schedule 3 drugs have a moderate potential for abuse and dependency, relative to the other scheduled drugs.

Phendimetrazine was FDA-approved in 1976. Currently, I would not say that this medication is as frequently prescribed as are the Schedule 4 weight loss medications.

#10 Phentermine (Adipex-P)

Phentermine is a sympathomimetic amine anorectic. It is a Schedule 4 controlled substance, meaning it has low potential for abuse (relative to Schedule 3 drugs). It was FDA-approved in 1959.

Phentermine is arguably the most widely prescribed weight loss medicine in the US.

It is prescribed as a single medication (off-label when taken long-term) or in combination with other drugs - both off label **(see the earlier discussion about Phen-Pro)** and as part of the brand-name drug Qsymia (see below).

Phentermine has a 55+ year history of relatively safe use (don't blame Phentermine for the Fen-Phen catastrophe! see the chapter *Phentermine; Guilty by Association*).

Phentermine has never been recalled from the US market, it has no black box warnings, and is currently being paired with other medications for FDA-approved, long-term (even life-long) use.

Additionally, it is inexpensive compared to other medications used for weight loss. For all of these reasons, Phentermine is central to obesity treatment for many, if not most bariatricians.

#11 Qsymia (Phentermine/Topiramate ER)

Qysmia is a combination of the two drugs Phentermine and Topiramate ER. It is a Schedule 4 controlled substance (because Phentermine is a Schedule 4 drug; Topiramate is not scheduled), meaning it has low potential for abuse (relative to Schedule 3 drugs).

Qysmia was FDA-approved in 2012 for long-term (potentially life-long) use.

Phentermine is a widely used Schedule 4 sympathomimetic amine anorectic (see its details above).

Topiramate (Topamax) is FDA-approved as an anticonvulsant drug for treating seizures, but has been used off-label for weight loss for many years (**see *FDA-Approved Meds Used Off-Label for Weight Loss***). The specific mechanism of how Topiramate leads to weight loss is not yet known.

More details about each medication is provided separately.

Qsymia has a **WARNING**, a portion of which states:

Qsymia carries a risk for birth defects (cleft lip with or without cleft palate) in infants exposed during the first trimester of pregnancy (Topiramate has this risk).

Women who are pregnant, or are thinking of becoming pregnant should not take Qsymia. Women who can become pregnant should have a negative pregnancy test before taking Qsymia and should use effective birth control while taking Qsymia.

Additionally, Qsymia can increase the risk of suicidal thoughts or behavior (Topiramate has this risk), and can increase heart rate (Phentermine has this risk).

FOR THE COMPLETE WARNING VISIT:

www.Qsymia.com

FDA-APPROVED MEDICATION USED OFF-LABEL FOR WEIGHT LOSS

*T*here are 4 FDA-approved medications that are commonly used off-label for weight loss. They are listed in alphabetical order below and discussed in detail.

#1 Bupropion (Wellbutrin)

Bupropion is an antidepressant medication of the aminoketone class. It was FDA-approved in 1985 to treat depression and in 1997 for smoking cessation. It is not a Scheduled medication (not a controlled substance).

Bupropion is known to have a side effect of weight loss, so it is used off-label for this purpose.

Bupropion is one of the drugs in the combination medication Contrave which was FDA-approved in 2014 for long-term (potentially life-long) weight loss and weight management (see the chapter *FDA-Approved Weight Loss Meds, Combo Meds, and Meds for Longterm Use*).

Bupropion has a **BLACK BOX WARNING,** a portion of which states:

Antidepressants have an increased risk of suicidal thoughts and behavior change associated with their use. Additionally, serious neuropsychiatric events have occurred in patients taking Bupropion for smoking cessation.

FOR THE COMPLETE BLACK BOX WARNING VISIT:

www.FDA.gov

~

#2 Metformin (Glucophage)

Metformin is an anti-hyperglycemic medication and the first-line medication used in the treatment of type 2 diabetes. It was FDA-approved in 1994. It is not a Scheduled medication (not a controlled substance).

Metformin is often prescribed off-label for (modest) weight loss and diabetes *prevention*. It is taken before meals and works by reducing glucose absorption in the intestines, decreasing glucose production in the liver, increasing insulin sensitivity, and increasing glucose uptake in muscle.

Because of Metformin's unique mode of action in reducing blood glucose without altering levels of insulin, there is a very low risk of hypoglycemia.

#3 Naltrexone, low dose (LDN)

Naltrexone is an opiate antagonist which treats opioid dependency and alcohol dependency. It was FDA-approved in 1984. It is not a Scheduled medication (not a controlled substance).

Naltrexone is prescribed off-label in low-doses, often referred to as low-dose Naltrexone therapy (LDN) for several conditions, one of which is weight loss. How Naltrexone leads to weight loss is not yet understood.

Naltrexone is one of the two medications that make up the combination drug Contrave which was FDA-approved in 2014 for long-term (potentially life-long) weight loss and weight management (see the chapter *FDA-Approved Weight Loss Meds, Combo Meds, and Meds for Longterm Use*).

#4 Topiramate (Topamax)

Topiramate is an anticonvulsant medicine that has been prescribed off-label for weight loss for many years. It was FDA-approved in 1996 for seizure prevention, then approved for prevention of migraine headaches in 2004.

Topiramate is one component of the combination weight loss

medication Qysmia (see the chapter *FDA-Approved Weight Loss Meds, Combo Meds, and Meds for Longterm Use*), which was FDA-approved in 2012 for long-term (even life-long) use.

Topiramate is not a scheduled medication. It has been known for many years to have a side effect of weight loss, although it is not known how it produces this effect.

Topiramate has a **WARNING**, a portion of which states:

It carries a risk for birth defects (cleft lip with or without cleft palate) in infants exposed during the first trimester of pregnancy. Women who are pregnant, or are thinking of becoming pregnant should not take Topiramate. Women who can become pregnant should have a negative pregnancy test before taking Topiramate and should use effective birth control while taking Topiramate. Additionally, Topiramate can increase the risk of suicidal thoughts or behavior.

FOR THE COMPLETE WARNING VISIT:

www.Topamax.com

~

Bonus Drug: Phentermine (Adipex-P)

Yes. Phentermine.

As mentioned elsewhere in this book, technically when Phentermine is prescribed for beyond 12 weeks it is considered as being prescribed *off label* (don't be surprised if even your doctor isn't aware of this).

See previous chapters for details and discussions regarding Phentermine.

*NEW IN 2019 - FDA-APPROVED ORAL WEIGHT MANAGEMENT DEVICE

A prescription weight management device called *Plenity* was FDA-approved in 2019.

Rather than a drug, Plenity is classified as a *transient, space occupying device*. But don't let the terminology scare you. This novel prescription weight management aid is worth learning about. Read on.

~

What is Plenity and how does it work?

Plenity is a non-systemic, non-stimulant, superabsorbent hydrogel. It comes in a capsule and is taken by mouth with water before meals. The capsule releases thousands of particles of naturally-derived substances called cellulose and citric acid in the stomach. The particles quickly absorb water and expand to form a hydrogel which fills about 1/4 of the stomach.

The hydrogel increases the volume of the stomach and small intestine which produces a sense of fullness and satiety without adding additional calories, all of which contributes to weight loss. The gel passes through the digestive system without being absorbed into the bloodstream. The water from the gel is reabsorbed in the large intestine and the remaining gel is eliminated in the stool.

Plenity was approved for use in conjunction with diet and exercise. It can be taken alongside other weight-loss medication.

Criteria for treatment (*the best part!*)

Overweight and obese patients with a BMI of 25-40 qualify to be considered for treatment with Plenity. This is a significant improvement in the field of treatment for overweight patients because most prescription weight-loss medications are available only to patients with a BMI of 30 and up *or* to those with a BMI of 27-29 *if they also have other weight-related disorders such as type 2 diabetes, high blood pressure, or abnormal cholesterol levels.*

This is good news!

Because now patients with a BMI as low as 25 who have no *qualifying medical conditions* other than being overweight can be considered for treatment with Plenity.

This broader inclusion can potentially help millions of overweight (*and overlooked*) patients who were previously lost in the 'treatment gap' due to either having a BMI of 25-26 or by having a BMI of 27-29 but without additional qualifying medical conditions.

Is Plenity effective?

About 60% of adults treated with Plenity lost an average of 10% of their weight within 6 months. The weight management aid was reportedly safe and well-tolerated in clinical studies. The most common side effects were gastrointestinal symptoms.

Duration of use

There is no restriction on how long Plenity can be used to assist in weight management.

Availability and Pricing

Plenity is not expected to be available to the general public until 2020. Pricing information is not yet available.

Safety

Plenity should not be used by pregnant women. People with esophageal abnormalities or strictures or those with complications due to previous surgeries of the gastrointestinal tract should not use Plenity. People with active gastrointestinal issues and those taking certain prescription medication should use caution. People who are allergic to the Plenity's contents should not use it.

For more information about Plenity visit: myplenity.com

TESTIMONIAL ~ METABOLIC SYNDROME ~ WHAT IT IS AND HOW ORLANDO REVERSED IT

Metabolic syndrome is a life-threatening, obesity-related condition that is made up of three or more metabolic risk factors (listed below).

Having just one of these risk factors increases the risk of heart disease, stroke, and other forms of disease. The greater number of risk factors a person has, the greater their risk of medical devastation.

Other names for metabolic syndrome include dysmetabolic syndrome, obesity syndrome, insulin resistance syndrome, and syndrome X.

Metabolic syndrome is diagnosed when three or more of the following risk factors are present:

- Elevated blood pressure (or a person on medication for high blood pressure).
- Elevated fasting blood sugar, or a diagnosis of type 2 diabetes (or a person on medication for high blood sugar).
- Elevated triglycerides (or a person on medication for high triglycerides). Triglycerides are a type of fat in the blood.
- Low HDL (high-density lipoprotein) cholesterol (or a person on medication for low HDL). HDL is healthy cholesterol that helps prevent plaque from building up in arteries. So as a vascular-*protective* cholesterol, having low levels of HDL *increases* the risk of heart disease, stroke, and of other vascular disease.
- Abdominal (or *central*) obesity. This is the person with the large waistline or *apple* shape. For women, this would involve having a waist circumference of at least 35 inches around when measured from hip bone to hip bone with a tape measure, and at least 40 inches around for men. The increased risk is due to having excess deep, or *visceral* fat which is more dangerous than the fat that we grab when we 'pinch an inch.' Visceral fat is stored deep around internal organs. It releases chemicals that lead to inflammation and it also alters hormone level. Excess visceral fat increases the risk of type 2 diabetes, heart disease, stroke, and several cancers including colon, esophageal, and pancreatic cancer, and other diseases.

Because of the increasing rate of obesity, the incidence of metabolic syndrome is increasing as well. According to the NIH (National Institutes of Health) metabolic syndrome may surpass smoking as the leading risk of heart disease.

Fortunately, it's possible to prevent and reverse metabolic syndrome risk factors with healthy lifestyle changes, such as losing weight, improving our dietary intake, and incorporating moderate exercise into our daily lives.

Studies have shown that high-carbohydrate diets (60% of dietary intake or greater) result in metabolic syndrome risk factors. Insulin resistance, type 2 diabetes, high triglyceride levels, and low HDL levels are all associated with high-carbohydrate diets.

Additionally, carbohydrates can lead to the transformation of LDL (low-density lipoprotein) to VLDL (very low-density lipoprotein), which is a greater contributor to atherosclerosis (plaque build-up in the arteries), heart disease, and stroke than LDL.

Thus, restricting overall dietary carbohydrate intake is effective in reducing the symptoms of metabolic syndrome.

~

How Orlando Reversed Metabolic Syndrome

Orlando came to me for weight loss and was shocked to learn he had metabolic syndrome. Although he had a history of hypertension, prediabetes, low HDL, and central obesity, his doctor had never discussed having metabolic syndrome with him nor had he ever heard of it.

After discussing the syndrome, its implications, and management, I prescribed medication for Orlando's high blood pressure.

Once his blood pressure better controlled, he was able to take prescription weight loss medicine, which I prescribed to help reduce his cravings for carbohydrates and to help suppress his appetite.

I counseled Orlando on the benefits of reducing carbohydrates (particularly sugary, starchy, and processed carbs) as this is the best dietary regimen to help reverse metabolic syndrome.

We discussed the importance of beginning immediately to make improvements in his lifestyle. Even if he could only start by taking small steps initially, a commitment to applying his best effort every day was most important.

Orlando was determined to improve his health and he accepted the recommendations wholeheartedly.

Over the following months, Orlando was slow to adopt exercise as a habit. He walked 30 minutes a day, twice a week to start, then slowly increased to four or five days per week.

He confessed that he "didn't eat perfectly," but he purposed himself to reduce his carbohydrate intake the best he could most days, keeping his goal of reversing metabolic syndrome in mind.

Orlando lost over 30 pounds in his first 60 days, and just over 40 pounds in four months. This was through Thanksgiving and Christmas no less!

Orlando's blood pressure and cholesterol levels completely normalized and we were able to discontinue his blood pressure medicine.

Although his blood sugar and weight had decreased, these were still above normal. But Orlando wasn't discouraged.

The lifestyle he had adopted was effective enough to have reversed metabolic syndrome and he couldn't be happier!

Orlando thanked me and let me know that he could take it from there. He enjoyed his new lifestyle and felt confident that he would continue along the path of healthier living. He no longer required additional counseling, nor any help from weight loss medication.

Orlando is a great example of what NMD is all about! Immediately striving to adopt a healthier mindset, taking action steps right away (See the chapter *Start Today. Always Today!*), and progressing daily as we are able. That's it!

We don't worry about how fast or slow we're moving, just as long as we stay in motion. Because even the smallest steps taken on a daily basis will eventually lead us to our destination.

How do you eat an elephant?

One bite at a time.

THANK YOU!

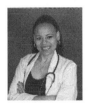

Thank you for reading *No More Dieting!*

If you benefited from this book, would you be a big help to myself and to others by leaving a review on the website from which you ordered this book?

Would you also share *No More Dieting!* on your social media pages? Thank you for spreading the word!

Feel free to contact me if you have any thoughts or suggestions you'd like to share. I'd love to hear from you!

Email: Info@NoMoreDieting.com

My very best to you!

Dr. Shauna Collins

ABOUT DR. SHAUNA COLLINS

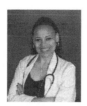

Dr. Shauna Collins is a physician, speaker, author, and medical researcher. She earned a medical degree from David Geffen School of Medicine at UCLA (formally UCLA School of Medicine), graduated Kaiser Permanente Family Medicine Residency and holds a bachelor's degree in biology with cellular and molecular emphasis from Occidental College.

As a specialist in bariatric medicine, Dr. Collins has counseled and treated over 1000 overweight and obese patients. Having overcome a lifetime of obesity herself, she practices from a unique place of knowledge, understanding, and compassion.

Dr. Collins is no longer in private practice, but travels full-time as a contracted medical researcher for the Centers for Disease Control and Prevention (CDC)-National Center for Health Statistics (NCHS). She has been recognized in television, radio, and print for her life achievements. But, according to Dr. Collins her greatest accomplishments are in caring for her family and inspiring others to design and live their best life.

For more information visit: www.ShaunaCollinsMD.com

Contact: Info@ShaunaCollinsMD.com

Made in the USA
Middletown, DE
09 September 2020

18755284R00102